# Current Topics in Microbiology and Immunology

159

Editors

# Immunological Memory

Edited by
D. Gray and J. Sprent

With 38 Figures

Springer-Verlag
Berlin Heidelberg New York
London Paris Tokyo Hong Kong

DAVID GRAY Ph.D.

Basel Institute for Immunology
Grenzacherstr. 487, CH-4005 Basel

JONATHAN SPRENT M.B., B.S., Ph.D.

Member, Dept. of immunology–IMM4A
Research Inst. of Scripps Clinic
10666 North Torrey Pines Road
La Jolla, CA 92037, USA

**ISBN-13: 978-3-642-75246-9** **e-ISBN-13: 978-3-642-75244-5**
**DOI: 10.1007/978-3-642-75244-5**


Softcover reprint of the hardcover 1st edition 1990
Library of Congress Catalog Card Number 15-12910



Phototypesetting: Thomson Press (India) Ltd, New Delhi
Offsetprinting: Saladruck, Berlin; Bookbinding: B. Helm, Berlin
2123/3020-543210–Printed on acid-free paper.

# Preface

Although immunologists know rather a lot about the manifestation of immunological memory, an understanding of the mechanism of memory at cellular and biochemical levels eludes us. Indeed, as we shall see, it is not even clear which of the several models used to explain the working of memory approximates to the truth. It is in order to report on approaches to this problem and on recent experimental advances in the field of memory cells that this volume has been put together.

In the past 4–5 years cell surface molecules that may enable us to define memory B and T cells have been identified. It may now be possible to ask how memory cells are generated and to define what signals are required during or after antigenic encounter for a cell to enter the memory cell pool rather than to terminally differentiate into an effector cell. The transition from virgin cell to memory cell is clearly accompanied by several biochemical changes. For B cells, isotype switching and somatic mutations (leading to affinity maturation) are well-defined phenomena, although the molecular mechanisms remain mysterious. Both have received attention in many excellent reviews of late and so are not considered in detail in this book. Neither switching nor somatic mutation is a feature of peripheral T-cell maturation; biochemical differences between virgin and memory T cells may only relate to differing activation requirements and possibly changes in the expression of accessory molecules.

A complete understanding of immunological memory, however, will come not only from the phenotypic definition of memory cells but also from studying how these cells maintain memory over months and years. The conventional model of memory has been that it is carried by a cell that lives for a very long time. If this is true, then one is faced with two questions. First, given that the majority of lymphocytes in peripheral lymphoid tissues have an intermitotic lifespan of only 4-6 weeks, how do memory cells alter their lifespan? Secondly, how do memory cells remove themselves from the selection pressures which shape the peripheral lymphocyte pool? One solution to the first problem is to postulate that memory cells themselves are not long-lived, but rather they self-renew to form long-lived clones.

There is still the problem of clonal selection: in a dynamic immune system self-renewal will require a stimulus. So, the corollary to the tenet that memory cells have the same lifespan as other lymphocytes but self-renew is that that they receive continual stimulation. If this model is taken to its logical conclusion, then we have to say that enhanced memory responses may be due not to the action of specialised cells but to the increased frequency of specific cells maintained by continual stimulation.

This model still has a problem; that is, what provides the continual stimulation? Two possibilities suggest themselves—antigen and idiotypic interactions. While even inert antigens can be stored over very long periods on specialised dendritic cells (follicular dendritic cells), the generation of anti-idiotypic antibodies or T cells may stimulate clones of cells long after antigen has decayed. Unfortunately the question of idiotypic interactions in long-term memory has received scant attention experimentally and so is not represented here.

The lack of experimental data, however, has not inhibited people from proposing rather different models for immunological memory. In its extreme form, the idiotype network theory predicts that memory need not be a function of single cells or clones but rather a property of the system as a whole (global memory). Thus, perturbing the network results in the formation of novel connections; these new circuits representing a "memory" of the experience. This is reminiscent of the theories of neural memory in which circuits of firing nerve cells called "cell assemblies" are seen as the basis of short-term memory. Long-term memory, however, would require continual electrical activity in the cell assemblies, just as idiotype–anti-idiotype interactions should persist if they are the basis of memory. It has been suggested that repetitive firing within the assembly causes alteration of the synapse, such that it becomes more efficient and enables a signal arriving at just one cell to trigger the whole assembly. Interesting though these parallels are, it is difficult to see how reinforced circuits could be formed in a disperse and dynamic lymphoid system. Indeed, there is little, if any, firm evidence for network involvement in immunological memory.

We have stressed in this short overview the importance of establishing how memory is maintained. The contributions collected in this volume address this question but also provide information about new markers for memory cells and the functional properties of subpopulations expressing these molecules. It is clearly not only important from a theoretical point of view to distinguish between the models of immune memory: finding a "solution" to memory might have profound consequences on the design of new vaccination programmes.

DAVID GRAY
JONATHAN SPRENT

# List of Contents

## List of Contributors

(Their addresses can be found at the beginning of their respective chapters)

# Expansion, Selection and Maintenance of Memory B-Cell Clones

D. GRAY[1] and T. LEANDERSON[2]



## 1 Introduction

What do immunologists mean when they talk about memory? At the level of immune responses this is not too difficult to define as there are several properties of a secondary (or memory) response that differ from a primary response, i.e. the kinetics of a secondary response are accelerated, the isotype of antibody produced is different (relatively more IgG or IgA compared with IgM) and the affinity of the antibody produced is increased. However, at the cellular level definitions are many and varied. Current convention regards memory B cells as long-lived, resting cells (HOOD et al. 1984) that have switched to isotypes downstream of $\mu$ and $\delta$ (COFFMAN and COHN 1977; BLACK et al. 1980), although many still express these isotypes (BLACK et al. 1980; YEFENOF et al. 1985; ZAN-BAR et al. 1979) while carrying somatically mutated V genes (BEREK et al. 1987; SIEKEVITZ et al. 1987) and having different activation requirements (YEFENOF et al. 1985, 1986; PILLAI et al. 1984).

To date we have not been able to identify phenotypically a single discrete population of B cells that carries memory. A minimal definition of a memory B cell would be a cell that has undergone an antigen experience but does not as a

[1] Basel Institute for Immunology, Grenzacherstrasse 487, CH-4058 Basel, Switzerland
[2] Department of Immunology, Biomedical Center, University of Uppsala, Box 582, S-751 23 Uppsala, Sweden

Current Topics in Microbiology and Immunology, Vol. 159

result embark upon terminal differentiation to the plasma cell stage. The means by which this "decision" is made is a central remaining question in this field. Is it a lack of appropriate T-cell factors that prevents a B cell from differentiating; does the site of antigenic encounter provide qualitatively different signals; does differentiation depend upon the sort of T cell available; could a negative signal be supplied (suppression leading to memory; SCHULER et al. 1984); or do memory B cells and primary B cells belong to separate lineages (LINTON et al. 1989; KLINMAN and LINTON, this volume)?

Many of the events and signals (or lack of them) that lead to memory cell formation occur in germinal centres. The work of KLAUS (1978), KLAUS and HUMPHREY (1977), KLAUS et al. (1980) and COICO et al. (1983) demonstrates the importance of these proliferating foci within lymphoid follicles in the generation of secondary immune responses. In the first part of this review we will consider the types of cells and types of signals available within these structures and also whether germinal centres are the sites of somatic mutation. It will become clear that the form and location of the antigen plays a central role in the decision not to differentiate to a plasma cell. In the second part we will consider the role that antigens play in the maintenance of memory B-cell clones, which leads us to ask if memory is only the transient increase in frequency of antigen-specific precursors and whether the observed longevity of memory is purely due to persistence of the antigen.

## 2 Microenvironments and Memory Formation

The generation of memory B cells appears temporally and functionally distinct from the production of antibody-secreting cells. This has led to the notion that these cells may be of a different lineage to that of primary B cells (LINTON et al. 1989; KLINMAN and LINTON, this volume). However, the observations made concerning generation of memory can be equally well explained by the proposal that the choice of differentiation to plasma cell or to memory cell is influenced by the quality of signal(s) that the B cell receives and/or the microenvironment in which it receives the signal(s).

There are no hard data at present concerning the signals that push a virgin B cell into the memory cell pathway. In other words, we do not know what makes a B cell enter a germinal centre, however, we do have information on the sorts of cells that can be stimulated by antigen in these sites and that may initiate such a reaction. It is possible to investigate the sites of activation of virgin and memory B cells in adoptive transfer experiments by infusing K allotype-marked cells from antigen-primed donors into recipients that have been irradiated while their hind limbs (20% of bone marrow) were shielded (GRAY et al. 1986; GRAY 1988a). Immunization of these chimaeras with soluble antigen results in activation of both host (virgin) and donor (memory) B cells; in contrast to the memory response, the host virgin response wanes after the first week (GRAY et al. 1986). This is in part due to competition with high-affinity memory clones as antigen levels fall (GRAY et al. 1986; GRAY 1988a). However, as antigen is relocalized during this time, as immune complex, onto follicular dendritic cells (FDCs; NOSSAL and ADA 1971; NOSSAL et al. 1968; HUMPHREY and FRANK 1967), it may also be due to differences in the migration patterns of virgin and memory B cells. The results of experiments by STROBER and DILLEY (1973) and STROBER (1975) originally suggested that virgin B cells were not part of the recirculating pool, and more recently LORTAN et al. (1987) showed that virgin B cells (bone marrow cells depleted of recirculating lymphocytes) upon adoptive transfer (into K-allotype distinct congenic rats) did not localize or home is into follicular structures within the spleen or lymph nodes.

Restriction of antigen to sites that are only available to cells of the recirculating pool results in very poor stimulation of host virgin B cells in irradiation bone marrow chimaeras (GRAY 1988a). Figure 1a shows that immunization with antigen–antibody complexes that rapidly localize onto FDCs within B-cell follicles does not effectively stimulate virgin (host) B cells, but does elicit a strong donor (recirculating cell) response. Likewise, antigen restricted to a peripheral lymph node (such that no antigen reaches the spleen) does not elicit a virgin response (Fig. 1b). Similar chimaeras immunized i.v. with soluble antigen show equivalent virgin and recirculating memory cell responses. The conclusion is that virgin B cells are activated outside the follicular structures (in the splenic marginal zone, red pulp or outer T zones) and that this is a requirement for entry into the recirculating pool.

Furthermore, it is possible to categorize these bone marrow chimaeras into those that show a primary but transient host (virgin) response and those that do not. On following the host responses of these animals, over a period of months the ones that showed a transient primary response later produced an increase in host serum antibody, while those that showed no primary response did not produce any host antibody without further immunization. This is despite the fact that antigen persists in these animals on the surface of FDCs and stimulates donor memory responses over the same period (GRAY 1988a). Thus, continued recruitment of virgin B cells does not occur once responses are established, as antigen is only found on FDCs. We can also conclude that cells that initiate a germinal centre reaction are cells that have been previously activated while outside this follicular site. We have provided evidence that virgin B cells do not enter the follicular microenvironment, or are not capable of being activated there. It is still not clear whether after activation, only certain subsets (memory cell precursors) initiate germinal centres or whether the signal to do this is qualitatively different from the signal that stimulates terminal differentiation. However, a third possibility is that the process is purely stochastic. If this is the case, some cells will develop into plasma cells while some cells, by chance, will arrive in follicles and receive signals from T cells or FDCs that induce proliferation. In the next section we will consider B-cell activation in terms of this microenvironment.

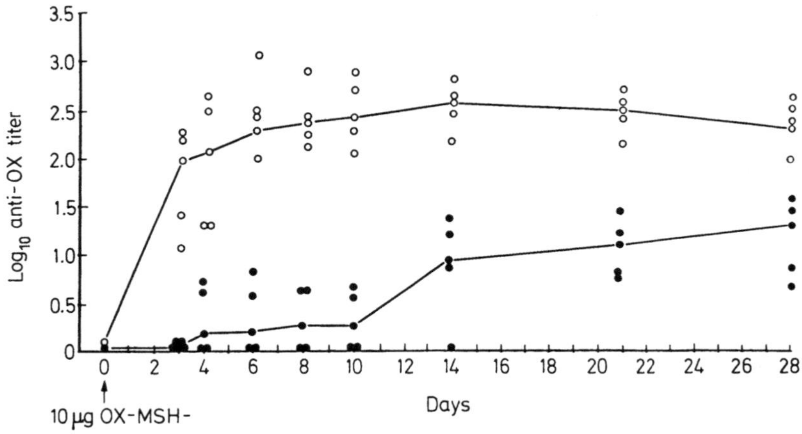


**a** anti-MSH complex

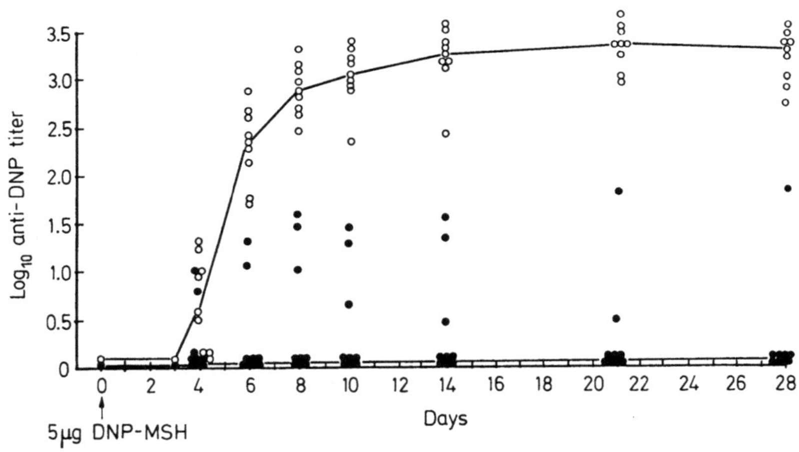


**b** in foopad

**Fig. 1 a, b.** Antibody responses derived from host virgin B cells and donor memory B cells in irradiation bone marrow chimaeras. **a** Anti-oxazolone antibody production of donor (○) and host (●) origin in chimaeric rats immunized with 10 μg oxazolone-haemocyanin complexed with antisera to haemocyanin (*ox-MSH-anti-MSH*)-, i.e. no antibody to oxazolone epitopes. Donors were primed with DNP-haemocyanin. **b** Anti-DNP antibody production of donor (○) and host (●) origin in chimaeric rats immunized with 5 μg DNP-haemocyanin (*DNP-MSH*) in Freund's incomplete adjuvant in front foot pads. No antigen reached the spleen at this dose as assessed by a plaque-forming assay. Each *circle* represents the serum anti-hapten titre from one animal. Lines are drawn between median titres. This figure is a composite of two figures from GRAY (1988a)

# 3 Signals and Cell Interactions Required for Memory Formation

Ideally we would like to investigate the interactions and signals that occur in vivo during the generation of a memory cell from a resting, virgin B cell. Although tissue sections may give some information about the proximity of cells, the only way to proceed appears to be to draw parallels with the data concerning B-cell activation, proliferation and differentiation in vitro.

The first step is the activation of the resting virgin B lymphocyte. This can be achieved by specific antigen and an interaction with an H2-restricted T-helper cell (KATZ et al. 1973; SPRENT 1978; ANDERSSON et al. 1980; SCHREIER et al. 1980). However, surface receptor cross-linking (with anti-immunoglobulin (Ig) antibodies), either alone (PARKER et al. 1980; DE FRANCO et al. 1982) or in the presence of lymphokines (HOWARD et al. 1982), suffices to stimulate resting B cells into clonal expansion. In vivo the relevance of the latter findings remains to be clarified, however, receptor cross-linking seems sufficient for the preliminary stages of activation of B cells in responses to certain thymus-independent antigens (FELDMAN 1972; DINTZIS et al. 1976). This initial phase of the response as we have seen (Sect. 2) occurs mainly in extrafollicular sites in secondary lymphoid tissues and may be transient due to the short half-life of antigen in these sites (FOSSUM et al. 1984; STEINMAN and NUSSENZWEIG 1980; MANDEL et al. 1980). Cell interactions that occur in vivo at this stage are not well defined. The initial activation of cells from cell cycle phase $G_0$ to $G_1$ and possibly beyond may proceed in the absence of T-cell signals (MELCHERS and LERNHARDT 1985).

The next step for the B cell in an immune response demands that a choice be made. The cell must differentiate directly into an antibody-secreting cell (probably IgM) or undergo clonal expansion in a germinal centre. As we have seen, the decision might be influenced by the site at which a signal is delivered, but it might also depend upon the stage of the cell cycle at the time of delivery. The degree of expansion that occurs in the initial in vivo IgM response, prior to the germinal centre reaction, is unclear but may be restricted to six or seven divisions of only 1 to $10^5$ cells (QUINTANS and LEFKOVITS 1974). The major clonal expansion that takes the response into its secondary phase occurs in the germinal centres. Here a selection of the B cells expanded during the initial phase of the response proliferate exponentially and extremely rapidly, having a generation time of about 7 h (ZHANG et al. 1988). Few of the cells exit the proliferating cycle to differentiate into plasma cells in these sites (STEIN et al. 1982). Only a minority of germinal centre B cells ever leave, either to differentiate or to recirculate as memory cells.

Are there any in vitro systems that mimic this proliferative response in the absence of secretion? In vitro exponential proliferation of B cells seems to require multiple signals, although these can be bypassed using mitogens (ANDERSSON et al. 1972; COUTINHO and MÖLLER 1975). Hence, anti-Ig antibodies together with various lymphokines (MELCHERS and LERNHARDT 1985; RAJASEKAR et al. 1988) or T helper cells capable of a cognate interaction with the activated B cells (RAJASEKAR et al. 1987) will induce proliferation. Mitogens or interactions with T cells always induce antibody secretion at one point during the culture. However, this terminal differentiation can be inhibited by addition of anti-IgM antibodies to the cultures (ANDERSSON et al. 1974; KEARNEY et al. 1976; LEANDERSON and FORNI 1984; HÖGBOM et al. 1987). This negative signal for differentiation operates even in the presence of lymphokines (RAJASEKAR et al. 1988) and is only relieved if a cognate T helper cell is provided for interaction (RAJASEKAR et al. 1987, 1988). Table 1 summarizes these regulatory requirements. So while proliferation continues, differentiation is down-regulated by a block at the level of transcription of the secretory form of IgM or indeed other downstream isotypes (LEANDERSON and FORNI 1984; HÖGBOM et al. 1987; LEANDERSON et al. 1987).

In the germinal centre there are certain parallels that can be drawn with the in vitro situation. Antigen to which preactivated B cells are responding is present in the germinal centres on the surface of FDCs, where it is in the form of an antigen–antibody complex and is bound via Fc or C3 receptors (HUMPHREY and FRANK 1967; PAPAMICHAIL et al. 1975). This non-processed antigen is presented to the B cells on a solid (cell) surface as repetitive subunits, such that cross-linking of receptors would be possible. Other immunoregulatory molecules might also be presented with antigen on the surface of these cells. We can only speculate about the production or localization of lymphokines by FDCs, but one molecule that has been found to play a role in the progression of B cells through cell cycle is the complement component C3 (ERDEI et al. 1985; MELCHERS et al. 1985). This is found deposited in the complexes on the FDCs and indeed is necessary for the initial localization of the complex (PAPAMICHAIL et al. 1975). Another important molecule in this microenvironment may turn out to be the low-affinity IgE Fc receptor or CD23 that is implicated in the growth regulation of human B cells (GORDON et al. 1989). What does seem to be lacking in the germinal centre is the presence of T cells. This absence is particularly apparent in the dark zone of the centre where proliferation is occurring, while in the light zone (where cells exit cell cycle) and in the small lymphocytic corona $CD4^+$, T cells are relatively frequent (NIEUWENHUIS and OPSTELTEN 1984). This may be the reason for proliferation in

**Table 1.** Signals and cell interactions required for B cell activation

| | In vitro | In vivo |
|---|---|---|
| Activation of resting B cells | Anti-Ig Cognate T-cell help (+ antigen) Mitogens (e.g. LPS) | ? |
| Exponential B-cell growth | Anti-Ig + lymphokines Cognate T-cell help (+ antigen) Mitogens | ? |
| Induction of high rate antibody secretion | Cognate T-cell help (+ antigen) Mitogens | Cognate T-cell help (+ antigen) |

the absence of secretion in the germinal centre as this last step in B cell differentiation is strictly T-cell dependent (SPRENT 1978).

Events that persuade a B cell to leave the germinal centre are not at all understood. This subject will be considered in the following section in some detail, but it should suffice to say here that in order to proceed to secretion (and possibly to survive as a memory cell) the B cell must find an antigen (carrier)-specific T cell with which to interact.

To elucidate the cellular interactions within the germinal centre we have begun to construct in vitro a similar microenvironment. Using FDCs enriched from immunized lymph nodes, preliminary results suggest that in the presence of these cells B cells proliferate directly from the lymph node. The proliferation is dependent on the presence of FDCs and T cells (KOSCO and GRAY, unpublished data).

## 4 Selection of Secondary B Cells

Somatically mutated Ig molecules are first detected during the 2nd week of immune responses (BEREK et al. 1985; GRIFFITHS et al. 1984; ALLEN et al. 1987; WYSOCKI et al. 1986). While it is not clear whether the process of hypermutation of Ig-V genes is an event that is only switched on during an antigen-driven response (WABL et al. 1987), it is probable that almost all somatic mutants are generated during the rapid clonal expansion that occurs at this time. In other words, the germinal centre might be the site where somatic mutations occur. There are two properties of germinal centres which make them ideally suited for this process. Firstly, the rapid proliferation of B cells in these centres (cell cycle time of 7 h; ZHANG et al. 1988) provides the opportunity for many nucleotide replacements to occur. Secondly, antigen is present on FDCs as immune complex, providing a mechanism for stimulating only those cells expressing receptors of increased affinity.

If somatic mutation is occurring within the germinal centres, these B-cell populations should also contain mutants of lower affinity and cells that have lost binding capacity altogether. If selection also operates at this site, the antigen non-binding cells should be found only in the germinal centre and not in the recirculating pool. To test this hypothesis we purified germinal centre B cells from the lymph nodes of mice undergoing a response to 2-phenyl-oxazolone (phOx) linked to ovalbumin (OVA). The purification was facilitated by the strong binding of the lectin peanut agglutinin (PNA) to these cells. $PNA^{hi}$ and $PNA^{lo}$ populations were fused and cell lysates from the resulting hybridomas were screened for expression of V genes commonly used in the primary response to phOx. $V_H$oxl and $V_K$oxl gene segments code for V regions that in combination form an antibody-binding site of relatively high affinity for phOx (KAARTINEN et al. 1983a, b), and these antibodies predominate in the primary response

(KAARTINEN et al. 1983b). We searched for clones carrying $V_H$oxl and $V_K$oxl in combination that had little or no phOx-binding capacity.

Analysis of several hundred hybridomas from PNA$^{hi}$ and PNA$^{lo}$ populations, taken 3 weeks after immunization, revealed not a single clone carrying $V_H$oxl and $V_K$oxl that had lost phOx-binding capacity. We found many $V_H$oxl/$V_K$oxl expressors in both PNA$^{hi}$ and PNA$^{lo}$ populations, but all had easily detectable phOx-binding affinities in radioimmunoassays. One conclusion might be that $V_H$oxl and $V_K$oxl gene segments in conjunction are capable of accumulating a large number of mutations before they lose their antigen-binding capacity (one antibody carries eight and nine replacements in the complementarity determining region (CDRs) of $V_H$ and $V_K$, respectively). However, stochastically one would still expect to find negative mutants somewhere in the B-cell pool (sampling of PNA$^{hi}$ and PNA$^{lo}$ effectively covers all peripheral B cells). The results at present do not allow us to conclude whether or not germinal centres are the sites of somatic mutation in B cells. However, the data do tell us something about the process of selection during an immune response.

Another conclusion might be that the lack of detectable $V_H$oxl/$V_K$oxl expressors that do not bind phOx is an indication of the stringency with which mutants are selected during the immune response. After all, if somatic mutation is a means of affinity maturation, it must be linked to an efficient selection process. We have postulated previously (MACLENNAN and GRAY 1986) that the mutating B-cell must obtain a signal via its antigen receptor if it is to survive in the recirculating pool. These results suggest that the mechanism of selection is so rapid as to preclude the rescue by fusion of mutated cells exiting cell cycle; it seems likely that progression through further cell cycles requires a new signal each time.

These data suggest that the immune system does not populate itself with redundant antigen non-specific mutants during an immune response. To date, four antibodies that have lost their antigen-binding abilities through somatic mutation have been identified (SIEKEVITZ et al. 1987; BRÜGGERMAN et al. 1986; MANSER et al. 1987). While MANSER et al. (1987) demonstrate no other indentifiable specificity for their antibodies, RAJEWSKY and colleagues show that one antibody (SIEKEVITZ et al. 1987; BRÜGGERMAN et al. 1986) has lost 4-hydroxy-3-nitro-5-iodo-phenylacetyl (NIP)-binding ability and gained anti-2,4-dinitrophenyl (DNP) activity. Both groups conclude that such antigen non-binding mutants survive and may have some function within the immune repertoire. Our data suggest that these workers were able to rescue by fusion a very minor proportion of the non-binding mutants generated during an immune response and that these normally do not survive for long, even in a germinal centre. In support of this interpretation, it should be noted that the two antibodies studied by the RAJEWSKY group were both selected during secondary responses following restimulation, not with antigen, but with an anti-idiotypic antibody that "sees" an epitope outside the binding site of anti-4-hydroxyl-3-nitrophenylacetyl (NP) antibodies.

In an attempt to mimic this situation we have been stimulating PNA$^{hi}$ and PNA$^{lo}$ cells with anti-$\kappa$ antibodies on Sepharose beads (plus supernative from an alloreactive T-cell clone) prior to fusion. Previous attempts to stimulate $PNA^{hi}$ B cells with anti-$\mu$ plus lymphokines and even lipopolysaccharide (LPS) + dextran sulphate all failed. However, anti-$\kappa$ on beads works efficiently, in agreement with data from LUI et al. 1989 that anti-IgG on sheep red cells prevents the apoptosis of human germinal centre B cells following overnight culture.

## 5 Maintenance of Memory B-Cell Populations

In the previous sections we have considered the central role of the antigen on the FDC in the expansion and selection of memory B-cell clones. However, antigen in this form is of continued importance in maintaining these memory cells over long periods.

The immune system has two options if it wishes to retain memory for months or years. The first is to have a subpopulation of cells generated during a primary immune response that have a very much longer lifespan than the majority of lymphocytes in the peripheral pool (average lifespan = 4–6 weeks; SPRENT and BASTEN 1973; GRAY 1988b). A second option is to maintain a record of all past immunological experiences by retaining antigens for many months or years. In this way both B and T cells could undergo restimulation at these depots. This would result in long-lived clones consisting of cells with a similar lifespan to most other lymphocytes.

Once the germinal centre reaction wanes after 3–4 weeks the B-cell follicle appears once more as a primary (resting) follicle; however, the FDCs around which the germinal centre formed remain an integral part of the follicular structure. Furthermore, they retain on their surface the antigen–antibody complexes that were localized here during the response. Antigens have been detected on these cells in the same native, molecular form 12 months after immunization (MANDEL et al. 1980). FDCs have been shown to retain more than one antigen (VAN ROOIJEN and KORS 1985), and so in effect they act as a library of the past antigenic experiences of the individual at a site through which recirculating B cells constantly migrate. The potential exists for continued stimulation of specific memory B cells by this antigen over long periods.

The consequence of continued stimulation should be the production of antibodies over a long period. In many cases this seems to be true; serum antibody responses elicited by soluble antigen in immune recipients or by antigen–antibody complexes are very long-lived (GRAY 1988a; MACLENNAN and GRAY 1986). Knowing that both antigen and immune responses are long-lived, it is important to find out whether B-cell memory is dependent on persistent antigen for its survival. Experimentally we determined, the lifespan of a memory B cell in the absence of any antigen. This was performed using $\kappa$-allotype distinct congenic rat strains by transferring $10^8$ $\kappa$1a thoracic duct lymphocytes (TDL) from primed donors (at least 2 months after the last boost) into lightly (500 R) irradiated κlb recipients. These cells were parked in the recipients for various periods prior to immunization. All chimaeras were bled and assayed for donor anti-DNP antibody prior to immunization; antibody production would indicate antigen transfer and so such animals would not be used. Figure 2 shows that the donor memory response rapidly becomes dominant if chimaeras are immunized 1 week following transfer. However, if immunization is carried out 3 weeks following transfer, there is a decay in the donor memory population. The decay is even more marked if immunization is carried out after 6 weeks, in which case the donor allotype response only surpasses the host response after 4 weeks, indicating that the donor cells no longer represent a functional memory population. When immunization takes place 12 weeks after transfer, no donor response can be elicited either with soluble antigen or with alum-precipitated DNP-keyhole-limpet haemocyanin (KLH) + *Bordetella pertussis*. The half-life of the transferred memory B-cell population in the absence of any antigen is around 1–2 weeks.

It should be pointed out that the normal in vivo situation is one in which antigen does persist for some time and if we transfer memory B cells together with

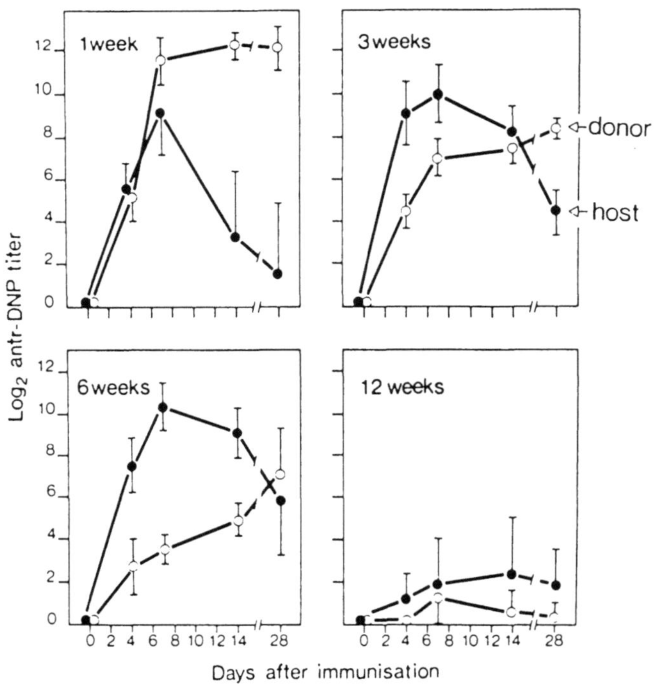


**Fig. 2.** The decay of memory B-cell populations in κ-allotype distinct adoptive hosts in the absence of antigen. The figure shows the serum anti-DNP responses elicited by i.v. injection of 50 μg of soluble DNP-haemocyanin from host virgin cells (●) or donor memory cells (○) in adoptive hosts at 1, 3, 6 and 12 weeks after transfer. The mean and standard deviation of responses in five to seven chimaeric animals is shown (*vertical bar*)

a small amount (5 mg) of soluble antigen the donor cells and secondary responses can be recovered 6 months after transfer (GRAY and SKARVALL 1988). So, memory B cells rely on periodic contact with antigen for their long-term survival. Does this mean that memory B cell clones consist only of activated cells? This does not seem to be the case, as both small, resting cells and large, activated cells taken from the thoracic duct of previously immunized rats (making high levels of serum antibody) will transfer memory to an adoptive host with equal efficiency (GRAY and SKARVALL 1988). It appears that following contact with antigen, memory B cells do return to a "resting" state but that in this state they have a lifespan of only a few weeks, in which time they must receive another antigenic signal. The importance of T-cell signals for the survival of a memory B cell is not clear. Certainly, once a B cell has met antigen, internalized and processed it, the B-cell must then find a specific T-cell in order to progress through terminal differentiation. However, the antigenic stimulus may be sufficient to act as a signal for survival and may explain why memory persists after antibody production falls below detectable levels. If memory B-cell clones are heterogeneous in size and activation state, it might be wise to be cautious about phenotyping memory cells until we know whether these surface markers are up- or down-regulated at different stages during the activation cycle.

## 6 Maintenance of Memory T-Cell Populations

The failure to evoke *host* as well as donor responses with soluble antigen in chimaeras 12 weeks after transfer of primed cells (Fig. 2) might be explained in two ways: by a lack of memory T-cell help or by a lack of the capacity to present soluble antigen to T cells. A third possibility is that of suppression, but this seems unlikely as it would have to occur only in chimaeras which have not been immunized; clearly no suppression operates if cells are transferred together with antigen (GRAY and SKARVALL 1988).

If the capacity to process and present soluble antigen to T cells was impaired then any memory T-cell help that survived in 12-week chimaeras would not be observable. Because the 12-week chimaeras retained no DNP-specific activated B cells, presentation to T cells might be inefficient (RON and SPRENT 1987). This was tested by transferring a small number of B cells from primed donors into 12-week chimaeras (GRAY and SKARVALL 1988). By doing this a host response could be evoked using soluble DNP-KLH, emphasizing the importance in vivo of B-cell processing and presentation of certain antigens to T cells (RON and SPRENT 1987; GRAY and SKARVALL 1988).

This result did not, however, rule out the possibility that memory T-cell help was lacking in the 12-week chimaeras. To test whether T-cell memory for an antibody response was also dependent on antigen for its survival, an experimental protocol to measure the decay of carrier-primed T-cell help in an adoptive host was used. This is shown in Fig. 3. In short, TDL from carrier-primed κla rats were parked in κ-allotype similar, 500-R-irriadiated recipients for 6 weeks and were either given 10 μg KLH or no antigen. At 6 weeks, $2 \times 10^7$ B cells ($4 \times 10^7$ TDL) from DNP-BSA-primed κlb rats wre injected into the chimaeras together with 50 μg DNP-KLH. This number of B cells produces a negligible response in the adoptive host unless it has been previously primed or given carrier-primed T cells; therefore, we assayed for the T-cell help remaining in the chimaeras at 6 weeks. Figure 4 shows that after 6 weeks there was a considerable decay in T-cell help in the chimaeras that received no antigen with transfer. One week after transfer, whether the animals had received antigen or not, responses were similar.

Accurate measurement of half-life of memory T cells in the absence of antigen requires more points on the curve. Surprisingly, the current estimate is shorter than that for memory B cells. This may reflect the importance of B cells in presenting antigen to T cells in long-term responses. Several weeks after immunization the only known deposits of antigen remain on the surface of FDCs (Mandel et al. 1980). As this antigen is not processed and is restricted to B-cell areas, the presentation is almost certainly carried out solely by B cells. The memory T-cell not only relies on the continued persistence of antigen for its

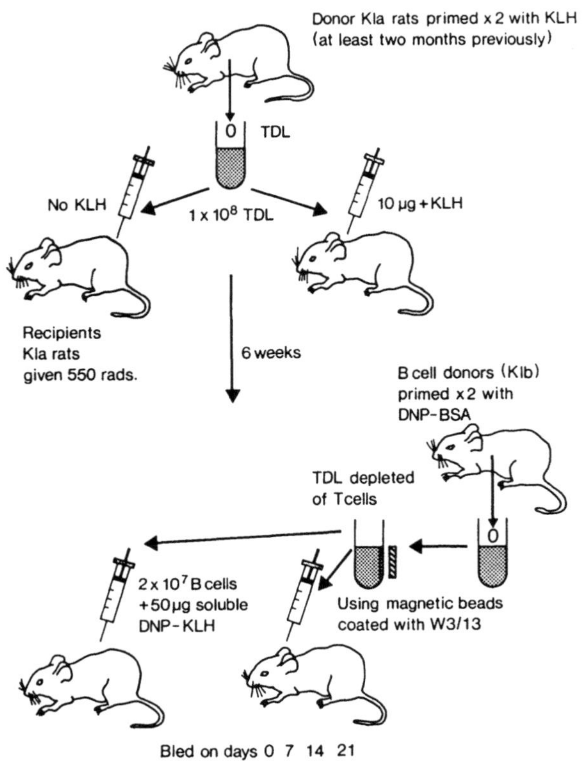


**Fig. 3.** Experimental protocol used to determine the longevity of T-cell memory in the absence of antigen

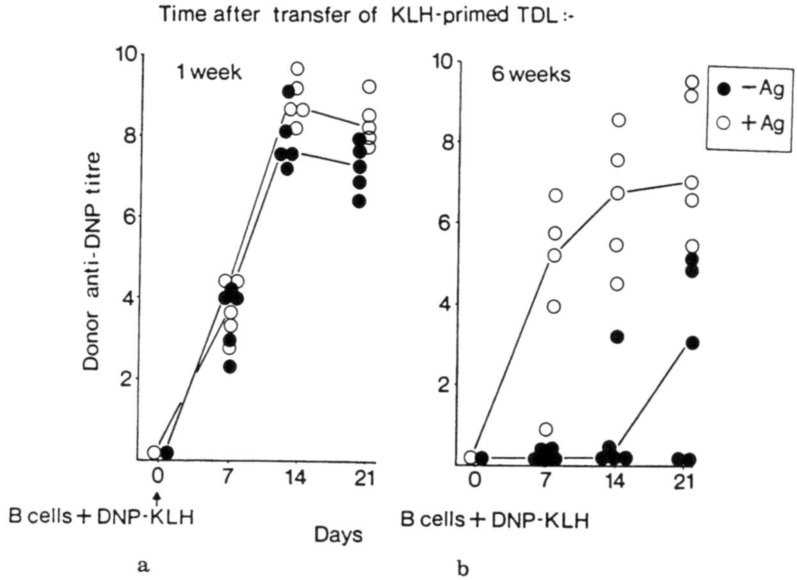


**Fig. 4 a, b.** The decay of KLH-primed memory T-cell help in adoptive hosts over a 6-week period in the absence of antigen. The ability of transferred KLH-primed T cells to help a limited number of DNP-specific B cells, following immunization with DNP-KLH, is compared in groups that did (○) or did not (●) receive 10 $\mu$g KLH at the time of transfer. Experimental protocol is shown in Fig. 3. Each *dot* represents the serum, donor allotype anti-DNP titre of one chimaera. *Lines* are drawn between median titres. *Ag*, antigen

survival but also on the survival of specific memory B cells in large enough numbers for a productive meeting to occur.

## 7 Conclusion

The pathway of generation of memory B cells from a precursor population remains unsolved. While the germinal centre is the site of expansion and selection of the secondary (memory) B-cell populations, the cells and signals that initiate the reaction are not known. We do have data to suggest that the precursor cell is one that is activated during the primary response prior to entry into the B-cell follicle. The important event in triggering the rapid proliferation that initiates the germinal centre reaction is the localization of antigen–antibody complexes onto the surface of FDCs. We feel that the B-cell proliferation in the absence of differentiation is related to the form of the antigen presented to the B cell on the FDC surface and the paucity of T-cell signals. The development of memory cells in preference to plasma cells may be a result of a stochastic process which depends on the migration of cells through this particular microenvironment. The process of clonal expansion seems likely to be accompained by somatic mutation. Whether this happens solely in a germinal centre is not clear from our data, but it does show that the selection against antigen non-binding mutants is very strong. The signal for survival and exit from the germinal centre seems to be received through the antigen receptor.

Signals received through this receptor are of continued importance in maintaining the memory B cell over substantial periods. We have shown that both the B- and the T-cell components of memory in humoral responses are short-lived in the absence of antigen. Their survival over long periods in vivo is dependent on the persistence of antigens as immune complexes on FDCs. Obviously some antigens such as viruses may persist at other sites. Memory does not reside with extremely long-lived resting cells, but rather with extremely long-lived clones that require continual contact with antigen for their survival. The longevity of memory in cytotoxic responses to H-Y (to which little antibody is made) is currently under investigation.

*Acknowledgements.* We would like to thank Drs. Claudia Berek, Uwe Staerz, Monte Wetzel, Fritz Melchers and Jean-Claude Weill for their critical reading of the manuscript. We thank Helena Skarvall for technical help and Nicole Schoepflin for typing. The Basel Institute for Immunology was founded and is supported by F. Hoffman La Roche, Basel, Switzerland. The work of T. Leanderson was supported by a grant from the Swedish Medical Research Council.

## References

Allen D, Cumano A, Dildrop R, Kocks C, Rajewsky K, Rajewsky N, Roes J, Sablitzky F, Siekevitz (1987) Timing genetic requirements and functional consequences of somatic hypermutation during B cell development. Immunol Rev 96: 5

Andersson J, Sjöberg O, Möller G (1972) Induction of immunoglobulin and antibody synthesis in vitro by lipopolysaccharides. Eur J Immunol 2: 349

Andersson J, Bullock WW, Melchers F (1974) Inhibition of mitogenic stimulation of mouse lymphocytes by anti-mouse immunoglobulin antibodies. I. mode of action. Eur J Immunol 4: 715

Andersson J, Schreier MH, Melchers F (1980) T cell-dependent B cell stimulation is H-2 restricted and antigen dependent only at the resting B cell level. Proc Natl Acad Sci USA 77: 1612

Berek C, Griffiths GM, Milstein C (1985) Molecular events during maturation of the immune response to oxazolone. Nature 316: 412

Berek C, Jarvis JM, Milstein (1987) Activation of memory and virgin B cell clones in hyperimmune animals. Eur J Immunol 17: 1121

Black SJ, Tokuhisa T, Herzenberg LA, Herzenberg LA (1980) Memory B cells at successive stages of differentiation: expression of surface IgD and capacity for self renewal. Eur J Immunol 10: 846

Brüggerman M, Müller J-J, Burger C, Rajewsky K (1986) Idiotypic selection of an antibody mutant with changed hapten binding capacity, resulting from a point mutation in position 50 of the heavy chain. EMBO J 5: 1561

Coffman RL, Cohn M (1977) The class of surface immunoglobulin on virgin and memory B lymphocytes. J Immunol 118: 1806

Coico RF, Bhogal BS, Thorbecke GJ (1983) Relationship of germinal centres in lymphoid tissue to immunologic memory. VI. Transfer of B cell memory with lymph node cells fractionated according to their receptors for peanut agglutinin. J Immunol 131: 2254
Coutinho A, Möller G (1975) Thymus independent B cell induction and paralysis. Adv Immunol 21: 113
De Franco AL, Raveche ES, Asofsky R, Paul WE (1982) Frequency of B lymphocytes responsive to anti-immunoglobulin. J Exp Med 155: 1523
Dintzis IM, Dintzis RZ, Vogelstein B (1976) Molecular determinants of immunogenicity: the immunon model of immune response. Proc Natl Acad Sci USA 73: 3671
Erdei A, Melchers F, Schulz T, Dierich M (1985) The action of human C3 in soluble or cross-linked form with resting and activated murine B lymphocytes. Eur J Immunol 15: 184
Feldman M (1972) Induction of immunity and tolerance in vitro by hapten protein conjugates. I. The relationship between the degree of hapten conjugation and the immunogenicity of dinitrophenylated polymerized flagellin. J Exp Med 135: 735
Fossum S, Rolstad N, Ford WL (1984) Thymus independence, kinetics and phagocytic ability of interdigitaling cells. Immunobiology 168: 403
Gordon J, Flores-Romo L, Cairns JA, Millsum MJ, Lane PJL, Johnson GD, MacLennan ICM (1989) CD23: a multifunctional receptor/lymphokine? Immunol Today 10: 153
Gray D (1988a) Recruitment of virgin B cells into an immune response is restricted to activation outside lymphoid follicles. Immunology 65: 73
Gray D (1988b) Population kinetics of rat peripheral B cells. J Exp Med 167: 805
Gray D, Skarvall H (1988) B-cell memory is short-lived in the absence of antigen. Nature 336: 70
Gray D, MacLennan ICM, Lane PJL (1986) Virgin B cell recruitment and the lifespan of memory clones during antibody responses to 2,4-dinitrophenyl hemocyanin. Eur J Immunol 16: 641
Griffiths GM, Berek C, Kaartinen M, Milstein C (1984) Somatic mutation and maturation of the immune response to 2-phenyl-oxazolone. Nature 312: 271
Högbom E, Martensson I-L, Leanderson T (1987) Regulation of immunoglobulin transcription rates and mRNA processing in proliferating normal B lymphocytes by activators of protein kinase C. Proc Natl Acad Sci USA 84: 9135
Hood LE, Weissman IL, Woods WB, Wilson JH (1984) In: Immunology, 2nd edn. Benjamin Cummings Merlo Park, CA, p 11
Howard M, Farrar J, Hilfiker M, Johnson B, Takatsu K, Hamaoka T, Paul WE (1982) Identification of a T cell derived B cell growth factor distinct from interleukin 2. J Exp Med 155: 914
Humphrey JH, Frank MM (1967) The localisation of non-microbial antigens in the draining lymph node of tolerant, normal and primed rabbits. Immunology 13: 87
Kaartinen M, Griffiths GM, Hamlyn PH, Markham AF, Karjalainen K, Pelkonen JLT, Mäkelä O, Milstein C (1983a) Anti-oxazolone hybridomas and the structure of the oxazolone idiotype. J Immunol 130: 937
Kaartinen M, Griffiths GM, Markham AF, Milstein C (1983b) mRNA sequences define an unusually restricted IgG response to 2-phenyl-oxazolone and its early diversification. Nature 304: 320
Katz DH, Hamaoka T, Benacerraf B (1973) Cell interaction between histoincompatible T and B lymphocytes. II. Failure of physiological cooperative interaction between T and B lymphocytes from allogeneic donor strains in humoral response to hapten-protein conjugates. J Exp Med 137: 1405
Kearney JF, Cooper MD, Lawton AR (1976) B lymphocyte differentiation induced by lipopolysaccharide. III. Suppression of B cell maturation by anti-mouse immunoglobulin antibodies. J Immunol 116: 1664
Klaus GGB (1978) The generation of memory cells. II. Generation of memory B cells with pre-formed antigen–antibody complexes. Immunology 34: 643
Klaus GGB, Humphrey JH (1977) The generation of memory cells. I. The role of C3 in the generation of memory cells. Immunology 33: 31
Klaus GGB, Humphrey JH, Kunkl A, Dongworth DW (1980) The follicular dendritic cell: its role in antigen presentation in the generation of immunological memory. Immunol Rev 53: 3
Leanderson T, Forni L (1984) Effects of $\mu$-specific antibodies on B cell growth and maturation. Eur J Immunol 14: 1016
Leanderson T, Andersson J, Rajasekar R (1987) Clonal selection in B cell growth and differentiation. Immunol Rev 99: 53
Linton PJ, Decker DJ, Klinman NR (1989) Primary antibody forming cells and secondary B cells are generated from separate precursor cell subpopulations. Cell 59: 1049
Lortan JE, Roobotton CA, Oldfield S, MacLennan ICM (1987) Newly-produced virgin B cells

migrate to secondary lymphoid organs but their capacity to enter follicles is restricted. Eur J Immunol 17: 1311
Lui Y-J, Joshua DE, Williams GT, Smith CA, Gordon J, Machennan ICM (1989) Mechanism of antigen-driver selection in germinal centres. Nature 342: 929
MacLennan ICM, Gray D (1986) Antigen-driven selection of virgin and memory B cells. Immunol Rev 91: 61
Mandel TE, Phipps RP, Abbot A, Tew JG (1980) The follicular dendritic cell: longterm antigen retention during immunity. Immunol Rev 53: 29
Manser T, Parhami-Seren B, Margolies MN, Gefter ML (1987) Somatically mutated forms of a major anti-p-azophenylarsenate antibody variable region with drastically reduced affinity for p-azophenylarsenate. J Exp Med 166: 1456
Melchers F, Lernhardt W (1985) Three resriction points in the cell Cycle of activated murine B lymphocytes. Proc Natl Acad Sci USA 82: 7681
Melchers F, Erdei A, Schulz T, Dierich M (1985) Growth control of activated, synchronized murine B cells by the C3d fragment of human complement
Nieuwenhuis P, Opstelten D (1984) Functional anatomy of germinal centers. Am J Anat 170: 421
Nossal GJV, Abbot A, Mitchell J, Lummus Z (1968) Antigens in immunity. XV. Ultrastructural features of antigen capture in primary and secondary lymphoid follicles. J Exp Med 127: 277
Nossal GJV, Ada GL (1971) Antigens, lymphoid cells and the immune response. Academic, New York
Papamichail M, Guttierez C, Embling P, Johnson P, Holborrow EJ, Pepys MB (1975) Complement dependency of localisation of aggregated IgG in germinal centers. Scan J Immunol 4: 343
Parker DC, Wadsworth DC, Schneider GB (1980) Activation of murine B lymphocytes by anti-immunoglobulin secretion. J Exp Med 152: 138
Pillai PS, Scott DW, White DA, Corley RB (1984) Major histocompatibility complex-restricted and unrestricted interactions in the T cell-dependent activation of hapten-binding B cells. Immunobiology 166: 345
Quintans J, Lefkovits (1974) Clones of antibody forming cells in pokeweed mitogen-stimulated microcultures. II. Estimation of the frequency of precursor cells and the average clone size. Eur J Immunol 4: 617
Rajasekar R, Andersson J, Leanderson (1987) Prolonged growth of activated B lymphocytes requires interaction with T cells. Eur J Immunol 17: 1619
Rajasekar R, Andersson J, Leanderson T (1988) Regulation of growth and differentiation of pre-activated B lymphocytes. Scand J Immunol 28: 509
Ron Y, Sprent J (1987) T cell priming in vivo: a major role for B cells in presenting antigen to T cells in lymph nodes. J Immunol 138: 2848
Schreier MH, Andersson J, Lernhardt W, Melchers F (1980) Antigen-specific T helper cells stimulate H-2 incompatible B cell blasts polyclonally. J Exp Med 151: 194
Schuler W, Schuler A, Kölsch (1984) Immune response against the T-independent antigen $\alpha$ ((1–3) dextran) II. Occurrence of B$\gamma$ memory cells in the course of immunisation with native polysaccharide is T cell dependent. Eur J Immunol 14: 578
Siekevitz M, Kocks C, Rajewsky K, Dildrop R (1987) Analysis of somatic mutation and class switching in naive and memory B cells generating adoptive primary and secondary responses. Cell 48: 757
Sprent J (1978) Role of H-2 gene products in the function of T helper cells from normal and chimaeric mice measured in vivo. Immunol Rev 42: 108
Sprent J, Basten A (1973) Circulating T and B lymphocytes of the mouse. II. Lifespan. Cell Immunol 7: 40
Stein H, Gerdes J, Mason DY (1982) The normal and malignant germinal centre. Clin Haematol 11: 531
Steinman RM, Nussenzweig MC (1980) Dendritic cells: features and functions. Immunol Rev 53: 127
Strober S (1975) Immune function and cell surface characteristics and maturation of B cell sub-populations. Immunol Rev 24: 84
Strober S, Dilley (1973) Biological characteristics of T and B memory lymphocytes in the rat. J Exp Med 137: 1275
van Rooijen, Kors N (1985) Mechanism of follicular trapping: double immunocytochemical evidence for a contribution of locally produced antibodies in follicular trapping of immune complexes. Immunology 55: 31
Wabl M, Jäck H-M, Meyer J, Beck-Engeser G, von Borstel RC, Steinberg CM (1987) Measurement of mutation rates in B lymphocytes. Immunol Rev 96: 91

Wysocki L, Manser T, Gefter M (1986) Somatic evolution of variable region structures during an immune response. Proc Natl Acad Sci USA 83: 1847
Yefenof E, Sanders VM, Snow EC, Noelle RJ, Oliver KG, Uhr JW, Vitetta ES (1985) Preparation and analysis of antigen-specific memory B cells. J Immunol 135: 3777
Yefenof E, Sanders VM, Uhr JW, Vitetta ES (1986) In vitro activation of murine antigen specific memory cells by a T-dependent antigen. J Immunol 137: 85
Zan-Bar I, Strober S, Vitetta ES (1979) The relationship between surface immunoglobulin isotype and immune function of murine B lymphocytes. IV. Role of IgD-bearing cells in the propagation of immunologic memory. J Immunol 123: 925
Zhang J, MacLennan ICM, Lui Y-J, Lane PJL (1988) Is rapid proliferation in B centroblasts linked to somatic mutation in memory B cell clones? Immunol Lett 18: 297

# The Generation of B-Cell Memory: A Working Hypothesis

N. R. KLINMAN and P.-J. LINTON



## 1 Introduction

The process by which secondary B cells are generated has intrigued immunologists for several decades. This is particularly true since appropriate antigenic stimulation leads both to a selective increase in the frequency of B cells responsive to the immunizing antigen and to the generation of a population of cells (secondary B cells) that are phenotypically and functionally distinct from primary B cells specific for the same antigen.

The basis for a few of the differences between primary and secondary B cells is now becoming well understood. For example, the ability of secondary B cells to respond rapidly by secreting antibodies of multiple isotypes and the expression of immunoglobulins of isotypes other than IgM and IgD as surface receptors (BLACK et al. 1977; TEALE et al. 1981) appears to be the consequence of heavy chain class switching (WAN et al. 1970; NOSSAL et al. 1971; PRESS and KLINMAN 1973; GEARHART et al. 1975). This process accompanies primary responses and appears to be greatly influenced by specific interleukins (MOSMANN et al. 1986; COFFMAN and CARTY 1986; COFFMAN et al. 1986; YOKOTA et al. 1988; FINKELMAN et al. 1988). On the other hand, the mechanisms that underlie many of the

Department of Immunology, Research Institute of Scripps Clinic, La Jolla, CA 92037, USA

Current Topics in Microbiology and Immunology, Vol. 159

phenotypic and functional differences between primary and secondary B cells remain poorly understood. These include the greater longevity of many secondary B cells (STROBER 1972; ELSON et al. 1976; MACLENNAN and GRAY 1986), the homing and recirculatory patterns of secondary B cells (STROBER 1972; MACLENNAN and GRAY 1986), the more rapid kinetics of antibody production and cell division upon stimulation of secondary B cells (KLINMAN et al. 1974; KLINMAN 1976; SIGAL and KLINMAN 1978; KLINMAN and LINTON 1988), the greater burst size of antibody-producing cell clones of stimulated secondary vs primary B cells (KLINMAN 1972, 1976; KLINMAN et al. 1974; SIGAL and KLINMAN 1978; KLINMAN and LINTON 1988), the relative ease of stimulation of secondary B cells with cross-reacting antigens (KLINMAN et al. 1973), and the relative inability of anti-idiotypic regulation to inhibit the stimulation of secondary B cells (PIERCE and KLINMAN 1977; OWEN and NISONOFF 1978; RAYCHAUDHURI and CANCRO 1985).

It should be noted that the functional consequences of many of these distinctions between primary and secondary B cells profoundly influence the outcome of primary vs secondary immunization. Thus, the relative rapidity, vigor, and longevity of secondary responses can be attributed not only to the availability of T-cell help and a higher frequency of B cells responsive to the antigen in question, but also to the aforementioned inherent differences in the parameters of secondary and primary B-cell responsiveness. In addition, the relative ease of stimulation of secondary B cells by cross-reacting antigens is one of the factors that helps to account for the phenomenon of "original antigenic sin," wherein secondary stimulation with a cross-reacting antigen generates more antibody to the initial immunogen than to the immunogen used for secondary stimulation (FAZEKAS DE ST. GROTH and WEBSTER 1966; EISEN et al. 1969; KLINMAN et al. 1973). Finally, the relative resistance of secondary B cells to anti-idiotypic suppression could play an important role in permitting B-cell responsiveness upon second contact with antigen in an environment suppressive for primary B-cell stimulation.

Recent studies by several laboratories have demonstrated that, superimposed on the differences between primary and secondary B cells, there is a rapid accumulation of somatic mutations in rearranged variable regions genes that appears coincident with the generation of secondary B cells (SELSING and STORB 1981; KIM et al. 1981; PERLMUTTER et al. 1984; MCKEAN et al. 1984; CLARKE et al. 1985; MANSER et al. 1987). Indeed, relatively little somatic mutation has been found, particularly early on, in the primary antibody response (BEREK et al. 1985; MANSER et al. 1987; SIEKEVITZ et al. 1987; MANSER 1987). Additionally, there may also be a paucity of somatic mutations subsequent to the stimulation of secondary B cells (SIEKEVITZ et al. 1987). Thus, the process of somatic hypermutation in immunoglobulin variable regions may be peculiar to the process of secondary B-cell generation. An important aspect of the somatic mutations that have been identified in the progeny of secondary B cells is that they appear to reflect a process wherein antigen has played a highly selective role. Somatic mutations appear to accumulate selectively in complementarity-determining regions and in nucleotides that affect amino acid expression as opposed to those that are silent. It is now believed that antigen selection of somatic mutations can help to account for two of the most characteristic attributes of secondary responses: (a) the relatively high affinity of secondary antibodies (EISEN and SISKIND 1964; KLINMAN et al. 1966, 1974; KLINMAN 1972; SIGAL and KLINMAN 1978; KLINMAN and LINTON 1988) and (b) the presence of specificities in secondary responses that are rare or absent in primary responses (KAPLAN et al. 1985; DURAN and METCALF 1987; JEMMERSON 1987). Thus, the presence of antigen during the generation of memory responses appears to play an ongoing role in the selection of (a) the highest affinity B-cell clones among those that respond to the antigen and (b) somatic mutations in responding clonotypes that result in more avid antigen–antibody interactions.

Among the proposed theories to account for the generation of both antibody-forming cells (AFC) and secondary B cells upon antigenic stimulation, the "unequal division theory" has been the most widely accepted (WILLIAMSON et al. 1976). This theory proposes that, by a process of unequal division, the progeny of stimulated primary B cells give rise to both AFC and memory B cells. The advantage of this theory is that repertoire expression is required in only one cell subpopulation to accomplish both primary antibody responses and memory cell generation. An alternative theory is that AFC and secondary B cells arise from separate B-cell subpopulations (KLINMAN et al. 1974; KLINMAN and PRESS 1975). The major advantage of the "separate lineage theory" is that it eliminates the need for a highly complex differentiative event, i.e., upon stimulation, a single B cell must give rise to daughter cells which differ from the parent cell as well as from one another. The generation of AFC and secondary B cells from different precursor cells might also be more consistent with differences in the kinetics observed for the generation of AFC and memory cells (KLINMAN 1976; WILLIAMSON et al. 1976). Perhaps the most attractive aspect of the separate lineage theory is that many of the differences between secondary B cells and primary B cells could be lineage specific and thus would not require complex differentiative events to yield secondary cells that differ so greatly from their putative primary progenitors. To date, the strongest argument against the separate lineage theory has been the inability to identify appropriate functionally distinct subpopulations within the primary B-cell pool.

Over the past several years, this laboratory has established procedures that permit the enrichment of two precursor cell subpopulations from the spleens of naive mice. One subpopulation, representative of over 80% of splenic cells, appears to give rise only to AFC clones, whereas the other subpopulation has the capacity to give rise to secondary B cells (LINTON and KLINMAN 1986; LINTON et al. 1988; KLINMAN and LINTON 1988; LINTON et al. 1989). Although we have not yet succeeded in the purification of these populations, the studies we have conducted provide evidence consistent with the separate lineage hypothesis. In addition, these studies have provided new insights into the parameters of secondary B-cell responsiveness that may help to unravel the complex set of interrelated events that account for B-cell memory.

## 2 The Enrichment of Progenitors to Secondary B Cells

A cell surface glycoprotein (Molecular Weight 48000) has been identified, through the use of the J11D monoclonal antibody, that is expressed at high levels (J11D$^{hi}$) on the vast majority of primary B cells but at low levels on the majority of secondary splenic B cells (BRUCE et al. 1981; SYMINGTON and HAKEMORI 1984). To ascertain whether relatively low expression (J11D$^{lo}$) of this cell surface glycoprotein might also be characteristic of primary splenic progenitors of secondary B cells, we separated spleen cells from naive mice on the basis of their relative levels of expression of the J11D marker. The J11D$^{hi}$ population of splenic B cells was enriched by subjecting the population of splenic B cells to fluorescence-activated cell sorting (FACS) and collecting the 40% of Ia-positive B cells that stained most intensely with the J11D monoclonal antibody. The enrichment of J11D$^{lo}$ cells was accomplished by pretreatment of spleen cells with the J11D monoclonal antibody plus complement, followed by the isolation of the remaining Ia-positive cells by FACS (LINTON et al. 1989).

To determine whether these two primary splenic precursor cell subpopulations differed in their ability to generate primary vs secondary antibody responses, $10^6$ cells of each population were transferred into lightly irradiated (400 R) major histocompatibility complex (MHC) syngeneic severe combined immune deficiency (SCID) recipients along with $2 \times 10^6$ purified $CD8^-$ T cells obtained from inguinal lymph nodes of syngeneic mice primed in the tail base with *Limulus polyphemus* hemocyanin (Hy). Within 2 weeks of immunization with 2,4-dinitrophenyl (DNP)-Hy, SCID mice repopulated with J11D$^{hi}$ B cells yielded a vigorous primary serum response, reaching a maximum anti-DNP antibody titer of 1 mg/ml approximately 3 weeks after immunization. After secondary immunization, these mice responded poorly, with antibody levels not exceeding those of the primary response and only slightly exceeding the levels in mice that were not boosted. In marked contrast, SCID mice repopulated with J11D$^{lo}$ primary splenic precursor cells mounted a relatively poor primary response that achieved maximum levels of 0.4 mg of antibody per milliliter at 2–3 weeks and dropped shortly thereafter. Upon secondary immunization, these mice responded both rapidly and vigorously, achieving serum anti-DNP antibody levels of 3.5 mg/ml within 7 days of reimmunization. Thus, the responsiveness of the J11D$^{lo}$ population of naive splenic precursor cells was consistent with the enrichment of primary progenitors of secondary B-cells since at least two immunizations were required to obtain vigorous antibody responses. Additionally, the J11D$^{hi}$ population revealed little in the way of memory B-cell generation and consequently showed little evidence of memory responses.

It should be noted that in order to observe the striking differences between primary and secondary responses in SCID mice repopulated with J11D$^{lo}$ precursor cells, it was necessary to inject soluble antigen in saline into one site and adjuvant into a different site. Since antigen emulsified in adjuvant is released slowly over several days, it is possible that the presence of antigen could coincide with the emergence of mature secondary B cells. If such cells are stimulated by residual antigen, their responses would appear to contribute to the primary response, thereby lessening the distinction between primary and secondary responses in these and other experiments.

To confirm these findings in vitro, we established a modification of the fragment culture technique which was intended to maximize the capacity for restimulation during the course of an in vitro immune response. Clonal responses in fragment culture are normally obtained by providing T-cell help through the use of irradiated carrier-primed recipients. It is assumed that, in such recipients, carrier help is provided by irradiated T-helper cells ($T_h$) present in the spleen that remain functional for a short time subsequent to irradiation. Since $T_h$ function could not be anticipated to persist for the 1–2 weeks needed to analyze secondary responsiveness in vitro, the fragment culture system was modified by the addition of viable carrier-primed lymph node $T_h$ along with the limiting diluted spleen cells. Control experiments demonstrated that the transfer of $T_h$ alone yielded no responses in fragment culture.

Our initial experiments using this protocol demonstrated that, if total splenic B cells were transferred, 80%–90% of total responses could be obtained upon a single antigenic stimulation at the time fragment cultures were established (day 0). Indeed, this protocol has been shown capable of the stimulation of 80% of antigen-specific cells that home to fragment cultures (Klinman et al. 1976) and has been used to enumerate cells responsive to a large variety of antigens in the fragment culture system (Klinman 1972; Klinman et al. 1974; Sigal and Klinman 1978; Klinman and Linton 1988). However, when nonirradiated viable $T_h$ were transferred along with the limiting numbers of spleen cells, restimulation between 7 and 14 days after initiation of cultures was found to generate an additional 10%–20% of clonal responses. The fact that the $J11D^{lo}$ population of splenic precursor cells was responsible for these additional responses was demonstrated in two ways. Firstly, when the J11D monoclonal antibody plus complement was added to the fragment cultures prior to primary stimulation, the majority of primary responses were eliminated while the majority of responses observed only after secondary stimulation persisted (Linton et al. 1988). Secondly and more directly, when B cells enriched for high levels of J11D expression were transferred into carrier-primed recipients, the majority of responses were observed after primary stimulation and few if any additional responses were observed upon secondary stimulation (Linton et al. 1988; Linton et al. 1989). Conversely, when B cells enriched for low expression of the J11D marker were used, only 20%–40% of the total responses were obtained after primary stimulation and the majority of responses were observed only after secondary stimulation. Indeed, the frequency of responding fragments was found to increase even after a third in vitro stimulation. Thus, consistent with the in vivo findings, the $J11D^{lo}$ population appeared to be enriched for precursor cells that gave rise to memory B cells whereas the $J11D^{hi}$ population was relatively devoid of memory cell precursors and included mainly primary precursors of AFC.

## 3 Affinity Requisites for the Stimulation of Primary AFC Precursors vs Progenitors to Secondary B Cells

Among the more surprising aspects of the aforementioned in vitro experiments was the finding that when fragment cultures containing J11D$^{lo}$ precursors were stimulated three times (days 0, 7, and 13 of culture), the overall frequency of responding fragments was two- to threefold higher than the total frequency of responses obtainable on a per B-cell basis from J11D$^{hi}$ B cells. This finding was consistent for responses to DNP, using cells obtained from BALB/c mice, and responses to (4-hyroxy-3-nitrophenyl) acetyl (NP), using cells obtained from C. B20 (Igh$^{b}$) mice. In one sense the relatively high frequency of responsive B cells in the J11D$^{lo}$ population is reassuring. As mentioned above, the vast majority of memory responses can be obtained when only 5%–10% of the B cells expressing the lowest levels of J11D are used either in vivo or in vitro, yet the overall frequency of secondary responses of total splenic precursor cells approached 20% of all responses. Since the frequency of responses among J11D$^{lo}$ progenitors of secondary B cells is at least twice as high as that of J11D$^{hi}$ primary B cells, the fact that 5%–10% of all precursor cells could give rise to 20% of the total responses is not surprising.

However, if the frequency of responsive J11D$^{lo}$ cells is uniformly higher than the frequency of responsive J11D$^{hi}$ cells, one might anticipate the stimulation of progenitors to secondary B cells to be less discriminatory and, therefore, less specific than the stimulation of primary AFC precursors. If this is the case, then the participation of a broader spectrum of clonotypes in the secondary response than in the primary response might be anticipated (for greater detail see below).

Perhaps the simplest explanation for the participation of a broader spectrum of clonotypes among stimulated secondary B-cell progenitors would be that the affinity requisites for the stimulation of these precursors may be less than those for the stimulation of B cells that give rise to primary AFC. If this prediction is correct, then clonotypes included in the primary B-cell response would also be included in the secondary B-cell response; however, the latter would also include clonotypes whose affinity might have been too low to permit adequate receptor–antigen interaction for stimulation of primary AFC precursors. Experiments are now underway to assess the relative affinity of monoclonal antibodies obtained from DNP- or NP-stimulated J11D$^{hi}$ and J11D$^{lo}$ precursor cells.

If repertoire differences between the primary and secondary B cells can be attributed to differences in the requisites of stimulation of progenitors of these cells, then disparities in the repertoires of responsive J11D$^{lo}$ and J11D$^{hi}$ spleen cells should be consistent with repertoire differences between secondary and primary B cells. To date, two experimental systems have been used to test this prediction. The results of both investigations are consistent with the interpretation that the secondary repertoire is, at least in part, reflective of the responsiveness of primary progenitors of secondary B cells.

In vivo or in vitro, the primary response of $Igh^b$ mice to the haptenic determinant NP is characterized by dominance of $\lambda$-bearing antibodies that are heteroclitic for analogues of NP with only a minority of the response being comprised of $\kappa$-bearing antibodies (which dominate most murine responses) (MAKELA and KARJALAINEN 1977; KARJALAINEN et al. 1980; KRAWINKEL et al. 1983; STASHENKO and KLINMAN 1980; RILEY and KLINMAN 1986). The secondary response of $Igh^b$ mice to NP includes $\lambda$-bearing antibodies; however, at the same time there is a considerably more vigorous production of $\kappa$-bearing antibodies. Using enriched populations of $J11D^{lo}$ splenic precursor cells from C. B20 mice, we have demonstrated that progenitors of secondary B cells, upon multiple in vitro stimulation, reflect the $\kappa$-dominance in NP responses normally characteristic of secondary B cells (see Table 1). Overall, the frequency of $\kappa$-bearing monoclonal antibody responses obtained from $J11D^{lo}$ precursor cells is approximately fivefold higher than the frequency in the population of primary AFC precursors (LINTON et al. 1989). Thus, the phenotype exhibited by $J11D^{lo}$ progenitors to secondary B cells is consistent with the phenotype of secondary B cells. The possibility that the high frequency of $\kappa$-bearing antibody responses is due to the recruitment of low-affinity responses is currently being investigated.

The second means by which the relative specificity of responses is being examined is by assessing the ability of cross-reacting antigens to stimulate the $J11D^{hi}$ vs the $J11D^{lo}$ cell subpopulations. As discussed in Sect. 1, one of the characteristic differences between primary and secondary precursor cells is the ability of secondary but not primary B cells to be stimulated by cross-reacting antigens. For example, we have previously published data demonstrating that, although the majority of DNP-specific secondary B cells can be stimulated in fragment culture by 2,4,6-trinitrophenyl (TNP)-Hy, few if any primary DNP-specific precursors can be stimulated by TNP (KLINMAN et al. 1973). To determine whether $J11D^{lo}$ progenitors to secondary B cells are, in this regard, more like primary precursors of AFC (i.e., highly specific in their stimulation) or more like their secondary B-cell progeny, which display considerable overlap in stimulation, we have initiated experiments intended to examine the ability of DNP and TNP to engender overlap stimulation in $J11D^{lo}$ progenitor cells.

**Table 1.** Responses of C.B20 splenic B cell populations to multiple in vitro, stimulation with NP-Hy

| Cell population | Stimulation with NP-Hy on days | Frequency per $10^6$ injected B cells | % $\kappa$-bearing cells | % $\lambda$-bearing cells |
|---|---|---|---|---|
| $J11D^{lo}$ $Ia^+$ spleen cells | 0, 8, 13 | 2.7 | 83 | 17 |
| Total splenic B cells[a] | 0 | 1.3 | 38 | 62 |

[a] Data from RILEY and KLINMAN (1985)

Preliminary findings indicate that, although only a small minority of J11D$^{hi}$ AFC precursors are capable of overlap stimulation by both DNP and TNP, a large proportion of J11D$^{lo}$ DNP-specific progenitors of secondary B cells appear capable of primary stimulation with TNP. Thus, the predilection of secondary B cells for stimulation with cross-reacting antigens appears, at least in part, to be a reflection of the response due to the J11D$^{lo}$ primary progenitors of these cells. The findings to date, both in the stimulation of $\kappa$-bearing NP-specific precursors in Igh$^b$ mice and cross-reactive stimulation of J11D$^{lo}$ precursor cells with DNP and TNP, can be interpreted as indicating the inclusion in primary responses of J11D$^{lo}$ secondary B-cell progenitors of specificities that would not normally participate in primary AFC responses.

## 4 Idiotypic Suppression and the Secondary B Cell Lineage

One of the more interesting differences between primary and secondary B cells is the relative inability of secondary B cells to be inhibited by anti-diotypic suppression (PIERCE and KLINMAN 1977; OWEN and NISONOFF 1978; RAYCHAUDHURI and CANCRO 1985). Table 2 summarizes some of the findings that led to this conclusion. It can be seen from the data presented in Table 2 that irradiated carrier-primed recipients that had also been primed with DNP suppressed over 70% of responses by primary Igh syngeneic splenic B cells, but did not suppress syngeneic secondary splenic B cells. The conclusion that this suppression is antibody and probably idiotype specific comes from the finding that primary B cells that are Igh allogeneic to the recipient are poorly suppressed. These experiments showed that, upon immunization, mice not only generate primary antibody responses and secondary B cells, but also develop the capacity

**Table 2.** Antihapten-specific B-cell responses in recipients immunized with carrier or hapten-carrier complexes

| Donor cells | Donor immunization | Recipient immunization | In vitro antigen | Percent response in Hy-primed recipients[a] |
|---|---|---|---|---|
| Primary splenic | None | Hy | DNP-Hy | — |
| B cells[b] | None | DNP-Hy + Hy | DNP-Hy | 29.5 |
| Secondary | DNP-Hy | Hy | DNP-Hy | — |
| splenic B cells[b] | DNP-Hy | DNP-Hy + Hy | DNP-Hy | 97.7 |

[a] This number represents the percent of positive foci detected in Hy-immunized recipient mice which were detected in DNP-Hy + Hy-immunized recipients
[b] From PIERCE and KLINMAN (1977)

to inhibit subsequent responses of primary B cells specific for the same antigen. The ability of secondary B cells to respond in these recipients seemed appropriate since secondary responses would likely occur in an environment wherein anti-idiotypic suppression had been established.

Recently, we have demonstrated that J11D$^{lo}$ progenitors of secondary B cells are also relatively resistant to the antibody-specific suppression. Among the mechanisms that could potentially explain the relative resistance of secondary B cells to antibody-specific suppression is the possibility that many of the idiotypes of secondary B cells may not be the same as those of primary B cells. This explanation may also pertain to J11D$^{lo}$ primary progenitors of secondary B cells whose responsiveness to DNP is also not suppressed in irradiated DNP-primed recipients. However, since it is likely that at least a portion of J11D$^{lo}$ progenitors to secondary B cells share repertoires with the clonotypes that dominate the primary AFC precursor cell pool, it is also possible that the progenitors of secondry B cells as well as secondary B cells per se are inherently resistant to anti-idiotypic suppression. In either case, the biological phenotype of secondary B cells in this regard, as in the other examples cited above, is reflected in the progenitor cell population of unprimed mice that appears to give rise to secondary B cells.

## 5 Tolerance in the Secondary B-Cell Lineage

As mentioned in Sect. 1, it is now known that somatic hypermutation plays a highly important role in the generation of secondary B cells (SELSING and STORB 1981; KIM et al. 1981; PERLMUTTER et al. 1984; MCKEAN et al. 1984; BEREK et al. 1985; CLARKE et al. 1985; MANSER et al. 1987; SIEKEVITZ et al. 1987). Since it may be anticipated that the process of somatic mutation could lead to anti-self specificities, it might be predicted that anti-self specificities that arise would likely be suppressed or tolerized during the generation of secondary B cells. To date, a high level of tolerance susceptibility has been found only to be a characteristic of immature B cells either from the spleen of neonates or the bone marrow of adults (NOSSAL and PIKE 1975; METCALF and KLINMAN 1976, 1977; CAMBIER et al. 1976; STOCKER 1977; TEALE and KLINMAN 1980, 1984). It is well established that mature primary B cells and mature secondary B cells are relatively resistant to tolerance induction even with high concentrations of tolerogens. We have now demonstrated that, like precursors of primary AFC, mature J11D$^{lo}$ progenitors of secondary B cells cannot be tolerized by the addition of appropriate tolerogens (haptens on carriers not recognized by primed T cells) prior to their stimulation in fragment culture. However, as early as 2–3 days following stimulation in fragment culture and as late as 8–10 days after stimulation in fragment culture, hapten presented on nonrecognized carriers has a marked inhibitory (possibly tolerogenic) effect on the subsequent responsiveness of the progeny of $J11D^{lo}$ secondary progenitor cells. Since this antigen-specific inhibition of the generation of secondary precursor cells can be inhibited with either free hapten or with hapten on the carrier used to prime the irradiated recipients and donor lymph node $T_h$, we have tentatively concluded that, during their generation, newly emerging secondary B-cell clones are highly tolerance susceptible. If this is so, then it would appear that antigen selection of newly emerging secondary B-cell populations may take the form both of positive selection for B cells expressing somatic mutants that yield a higher affinity for the selecting antigen as well as negative selection of somatic mutants that lead to anti-self recognition by newly emerging secondary B cells.

## 6 A Working Hypothesis for the Generation of B-Cell Memory

The identification of a subpopulation within the primary splenic precursor cell pool that appears responsible for the generation of B-cell memory has focused attention on the differentiative and selective events leading to the characteristics associated with repertoire expression in primary precursors to both AFC and secondary B cells. The clearest conclusions from these results concern the major population of splenic precursor cells that appears responsible for the bulk of primary AFC responses. Since these cells apparently do not give rise to secondary B cells, unequal division would no longer appear to be an issue insofar as these cells are concerned. However, our findings do imply that these cells, once antigenically stimulated, are not insensitive to the continued presence of antigen and the presumptive pressure of $T_h$ and the factors that they produce. Indeed, preliminary evidence both in vivo and in vitro indicates that, although these cells do not give rise to secondary B cells, antibody production by the progeny of these cells is prolonged by repeated antigen contact. Further studies of this phenomenon are now being undertaken.

Perhaps the most intriguing outcome of identifying a major cell subpopulation dedicated to the generation of primary AFC responses is the possibility that the process of somatic hypermutation might not apply to this B-cell subpopulation. As discussed above, it is possible to account for the appearance of somatic mutations relatively late in primary responses as the result of stimulation of newly generated secondary B cells by persisting antigen. Notwithstanding the finding of somatic mutants late in primary responses, studies of hybridomas derived from primarily stimulated B cells show a relative paucity of somatic mutations (Berek et al. 1985; Manser 1987). If somatic mutation does not play a major role in the generation of primary AFC responses, then the mysteries that remain with respect to repertoire expression in the major population of murine B cells would concern mainly the mechanism of V gene selection and rearrangement. Hence, primary B-cell repertoire expression would be largely established during B-cell development and tolerance would play a role only during B-cell development.

It would appear from the findings presented above that the burden for the generation of B-cell memory is carried by a small subpopulation of precursor cells within naive mice. Since this subpopulation is responsible for the generation of memory B cells as well as secondary antibody forming cells, defining a separate cell subpopulation responsible for the generation of memory does not necessarily obviate a possible role of unequal division in B-cell responsiveness. Furthermore, consequent to primary immunization, not only are antibody-forming cells and memory B-cells generated, but precursor cells that ultimately give rise to tertiary and quaternary responses etc. are produced. Since, in many instances, tertiary and quaternary responses build upon somatic mutations that accumulate after primary stimulation, it is likely that the progenitors to tertiary B cells are also engaged in primary and secondary responses.

Do the progeny of progenitors of secondary B cells then undergo unequal division subsequent to primary stimulation? The answer to this question is not yet clear; however, it may depend on how one views the process of differentiation and the meaning of "unequal division". One piece of evidence that may be significant is the finding that approximately 20%–40% of splenic B cells isolated as J11D$^{lo}$ give rise to DNP-specific antibody-forming cells after a single in vitro antigenic stimulation. This may imply that J11D$^{lo}$ progenitors to secondary B cells can also give rise to antibody forming cells. Alternatively, as will be discussed below, since the use of the J11D marker for enrichment of secondary progenitor cells is inefficient, some of the responses obtained from this cell population after primary stimulation might be accounted for by contaminating primary precursors to AFC. Additionally, any secondary DNP-responsive B cells that may be present in the spleen due to prior contact with cross-reactive antigens might also be J11D$^{lo}$ and would respond after a single antigenic stimulation. These responses notwithstanding, it can be concluded that the majority of J11D$^{lo}$ precursor cells isolated from the spleen of naive mice do not yield antibody producing cells after a single in vitro stimulation. Rather, at least two or more in vitro or in vivo stimulations are required to obtain antibody secretion from the progeny of these precursor cells.

The expression of differentiated cell clones which emanate from a self-renewing stem cell population in the bone marrow constitutes a form of unequal division common to the generation of a wide variety of cell types. If one views the mature primary J11D$^{lo}$ progenitors of secondary B cells as a potentially self-renewing "stem cell" population, then it is possible that this population, upon antigenic stimulation, could continue to renew itself while occasionally spinning off daughter cells which differentiate to form clones of secondary B cells. Since the progenitor cell in this case would already express rearranged immunoglobulin genes (they express cell surface immunoglobulin), somatic mutations could accumulate not only in daughter cells that become secondary B cells, but also in cells that maintain progenitor status.

Among the more interesting aspects of memory B-cell responses is the participation of specificities that are rarely, if ever, found within the primary response (KAPLAN et al. 1985; DURAN and METCALF 1987; JEMMERSON 1987). Indeed, although the secondary repertoire of a given individual may be relatively restricted, when considering responses of murine strains as a whole, secondary responses appear to include much of the diversity of primary responses (KLINMAN 1972; CANCRO et al. 1978) and may additionally include specificities not found in primary responses (CLARKE et al. 1985). This is particularly intriguing since the frequency of progenitor cells which give rise to secondary responses appears to be less than 10% of the frequency of cells that give rise to primary responses. In part, a more diverse repertoire in a smaller cell subpopulation could be accounted for by differences in the size and longevity of clones that express given clonotypes in the two subpopulations. It has been predicted from previous studies that primary B cells may be generated as clones of 200 cells (KLINMAN and STONE 1983). It may be possible that, in order to maximize diversity, progenitors of secondary B cells may be generated as smaller clones and cells of these clones may have a more rapid turnover.

Although these arguments could account for an equal expression of repertoire in primary and secondary B cells and may indeed help to account for the overlap of specificities in these two populations, these arguments would not account for the expression of specificities in the secondary repertoire which do not appear to exist to any great extent in the primary B-cell responses. In the above sections of this review, we have presented findings that indicate that this may be accounted for by the propensity of progenitors of secondary B cells to be stimulated by lower affinity interactions than those that are required for the stimulation of precursors to primary AFC. This was first observed by the finding that the frequency of responsive $J11D^{lo}$ progenitors of secondary B cells was higher for the DNP and NP haptenic determinants than the frequency of responsive $J11D^{hi}$ precursors to AFC. Furthermore, in addition to the normally dominant $\lambda$-bearing antibodies that are characteristic of primary responses to NP in $Igh^b$ mice, responses of secondary B-cell progenitors included a high frequency of $\kappa$-bearing cells which would not have been included in the primary responsive population. Similarly, many DNP-specific secondary B-cell progenitors displayed considerable overlap stimulation by TNP which is not the case for most primary AFC precursors. Taken together these findings indicate that, while no evidence exists showing disparities in variable region (V)-gene expression between progenitors of secondary B cells and precursors of primary AFC, elements of the V-gene repertoire that are excluded from primary B-cell responses appear to be included in secondary responses. This would enable the secondary repertoire to access a wider range of specificities which may include specificities that, upon somatic mutation, could result in high-affinity responses.

One highly intriguing outcome of the above considerations is the conclusion that the means by which secondary responses obtain their specificity may be quite different from the way in which primary responses do. In the absence of somatic hypermutation the total repertoire of primary specificities would be derived from germline genes and the product of their potential combinatorial associations. Tolerance and anti-idiotypic selection may dictate which specificities can be expressed as mature B cells. This conclusion is consistent with data demonstrating that, for a wide variety of antigens, the repertoire that is expressed in the primary B-cell pool of the adult spleen is entirely reflective of the repertoire as it is expressed from the developing surface immunoglobulin negative pool of the bone marrow (RILEY et al. 1983; KLINMAN and STONE 1983; FROSCHER and KLINMAN 1985; RILEY and KLINMAN 1986; KLINMAN and LINTON 1988). To date, all exceptions to this rule have been in the form of the occasional deletion of specificities which may be attributable to either tolerance (KLINMAN and STONE 1983; RILEY and KLINMAN 1986; MORROW et al. 1987) or network regulation (FROSCHER and KLINMAN 1985). Much of the specificity of primary antibody responses is therefore the result of a highly selective antigen trigger acting in an affinity-dependent manner on a diverse repertoire.

Secondary B-cell specificity, on the other hand, is derived from the availability of an even broader spectrum of potentially responsive cells which are stimulated in a much less specific fashion. However, in this case these specificities can continue to be selected in a positive fashion by antigens plus $T_h$ interactions or in a negative fashion by tolerance to self-antigens. In this sense, the specificity of secondary responses would result from a process that could be thought of as "somatic evolution."

Notwithstanding the finding that some progenitors to secondary B cells may be stimulated by residual antigen during primary stimulation, it would appear that much of the generation of secondary responsiveness occurs in the absence of the production of any detectable antibody. Thus, the generation of secondary B cells and the accumulation and selection of somatic mutants within this repertoire can be viewed as a phantom (silent) response that accompanies the more blatant responses (antibody production) of primary AFC precursors. Therefore, the early stages of secondary B-cell generation and the early events in somatic mutation would be missed by most analyses of serum antibodies or hybridomas produced subsequent to primary immunization.

## 7 Missing Links in Our Understanding of Memory B-Cell Generation

The identification of a cell subpopulation that may be responsible for the generation of secondary B cells has enabled the formulation of a working hypothesis for the generation of memory B cells. However, the data that has been obtained to date is far from adequate to permit any concrete conclusions concerning this process. As the data now stand, there are many crucial missing elements which render premature the drawing of any firm conclusions. Some of these uncertainties have already been mentioned in other sections of this review.

Our studies, to date, have utilized relatively few antigens and it is critical to know whether our findings would hold for other types of antigen, in particular, biologically relevant antigens. Similarly, it is important to determine whether the phenomena pertain to species other than mouse. In addition, it is not yet known whether other B-cell subpopulations such as the Ly1 B cells can give rise to secondary B cells. Moreover, the findings do not take into account previous findings by other investigators, i.e., those results showing that secondary responses may, with time, include J11D$^{hi}$ B cells (RAYCHAUDHURI and CANCRO 1985) and the unpublished work from the Sprent laboratory (J. SPRENT personal communication), indicating that memory B cells found in the lymph node are likely to be J11D$^{hi}$. Finally, all of our conclusions concerning the role of affinity differences in the triggering of primary AFC precursors vs secondary B-cell progenitors must be verified by affinity measurements of relevant monoclonal antibodies.

Most of the critical difficulties in defining a separate cell subpopulation responsible for memory responses could be resolved if an appropriate marker could be found which positively identifies precursor cells responsible for the generation of memory. To date, the only marker that has been available is the cell surface glycoprotein recognized by the J11D monoclonal antibody. Antigens recognized by this antibody are present on most bone marrow-derived cell populations and therefore are neither B-cell-specific nor specific for progenitors to secondary B cells. Enriching a population by the relative paucity of a given marker is at best a dubious experimental approach. Because of this, we have always assumed that most of our cell preparations, both J11D$^{lo}$ and J11D$^{hi}$, are cross-contaminated to varying extents. Most importantly, a proper marker could enable a definitive purification of the cells which give rise to secondary responses vs those which give rise to primary responses, as well as permitting an evaluation of the prevalence of such cells in various tissues and in various strains of mice of different backgrounds and antigenic experience. Such a marker would be essential for the establishment of secondary B-cell progenitors as members of a separate B-cell lineage.

Among the more intriguing of the above hypotheses is the prediction that somatic hypermutation may be confined to the B-cell subpopulation that is responsible for the generation of memory B cells. Whether or not this is true, and the stage in the life history of secondary lineage cells when somatic hypermutation is permitted, are experimentally approachable issues. We have already been able to establish hybridomas from SCID mice repopulated selectively with either J11D$^{lo}$ or J11D$^{hi}$ splenic progenitor cells, and the sequencing of these hybridoma antibodies indicates that somatic mutations do accumulate early in the course of secondary B cell generation from J11D$^{lo}$ precursors (LINTON et al. 1989). The demonstration of differences in the relative abilities of cells of these two populations to yield somatic mutations would not only further investigation into the mechanism of somatic hypermutation but would also serve as an additional and important marker for the delineation of disparate B-cell subpopulations and the characterization of B-cell memory.

## References

Berek C, Griffiths GM, Milstein C (1985) Molecular events during maturation of the immune response to oxazolone. Nature 316: 412–418
Black SJ, Van der Loo W, Loken MR, Herzenberg LA (1977) Expression of IgD indicates maturation of memory B cells. J Exp Med 147: 984–996
Bruce J, Symington FW, McKearn TJ, Sprent J (1981) A monoclonal antibody discriminating between subsets of T and B cells. J Immunol 127: 2496–2501
Cambier JC, Kettman JR, Vitetta ES, Uhr JW (1976) Differential suspectibility of neonatal and adult murine spleen cells to in vitro induction of B cell tolerance. J Exp Med 144: 293–297
Cancro MP, Gerhard W, Klinman NR (1978) Diversity of the primary influenza specific B cell repertoire in BALB/c mice. J Exp Med 147: 776–778
Clarke SH, Huppi K, Ruezinsky D, Staudt L, Gerhard W, Weigert M (1985) Inter- and intraclonal diversity in the antibody response to influenza hemagglutinin. J Exp Med 161: 687–704
Coffman RL and Carty J (1986) A T cell activity that enhances polyclonal IgE production and its inhibition by interferon-gamma. J Immunol 136: 949–954
Coffman RL, Ohara J, Bond MW, Carty J, Zlotnick E, Paul WE (1986) B cell stimulatory factor 1 enhances the IgE response of lipopolysaccharide preactivated B cells. J Immunol 136: 4538–4541
Duran LW, Metcalf ES (1987) Clonal analysis of primary B cells responsive to the pathogenic bacterium *Salmonella typhimurium*. J Exp Med 165: 340–358
Eisen HN, Siskind GW (1964) Variation in affinities of antibodies during the immune response. Biochemistry 3: 996–1008
Eisen HN, Little RJ, Steiner LA, Simms ES, Gray WG (1969) Degeneracy in the secondary immune response: stimulation of antibody formation by cross-reacting antigens. Isr J Med Sci 5: 338–351
Elson CJ, Jablonska KF, Taylor RB (1976) Functional half-life of virgin and primed B lymphocytes. Eur J Immunol 6: 634–638
Fazekas de St. Groth S, Webster RG (1966) Disquisitions on original antigenic sin I. Evidence in man. J Exp Med 124: 331–345
Finkelman FD, Katona IM, Mosmann TR, Coffman RL (1988) Interferon $\gamma$ regulates the isotypes of immunoglobulin secreted during in vivo humoral responses. J Immunol 140: 1022–1027
Froscher BG, Klinman NR (1985) Strain specific silencing of a predominant anti-dextran clonotype family. J Exp Med 162: 1620–1633
Gearhart PJ, Sigal NH, Klinman NR (1975) Production of antibodies of identical idiotype but diverse immunoglobulin classes by cells derived from a single stimulated B cell. Proc Natl Acad Sci USA 72: 1707–1711
Jemmerson RW (1987) Multiple overlapping epitopes in the three antigenic regions of horse cytochrome *c*. J Immunol 138: 213–219
Kaplan MA, Ching LK, Berte C, Sercarz EE (1985) Predominant idiotypy and specificity shift during the antibody response to lysozyme (abstract). Fed Proc 44: 1692
Karjalainen K, Bang B, Makela O (1980) Fine specificity and idiotypes of early antibodies against (4-hydroxy-3-nitrophenyl)acetyl (NP). J Immunol 125: 313–317
Kim S, Davis M, Sinn E, Patten P, Hood L (1981) Antibody diversity: somatic hypermutation of rearranged $V_h$ genes. Cell 27: 573–581
Klinman NR (1972) The mechanism of antigen stimulation of primary and secondary clonal precursor cells. J Exp Med 136: 241–260
Klinman NR (1976) The acquisition of B cell competence and diversity. Am J Pathol 85: 694–703
Klinman NR, Linton P-J (1988) The clonotype repertoire of B cell subpopulations. Adv Immunol 42: 1–93
Klinman NR, Press JL (1975) The B cell specificity repertoire: its relationship to definable subpopulations. Transplant Rev 24: 41–83
Klinman NR, Stone MR (1983) The role of variable region gene expression and environmental selection in determining the anti-phosphorylcholine B cell repertoire. J Exp Med 158: 1948–1961
Klinman NR, Rockey JH, Frauenberger G, Karush F (1966) Equine antihapten antibody. III. The comparative properties of the $\gamma$G- and $\gamma$A antibodies
Klinman NR, Press JL, Segal GP (1973) Overlap stimulation of primary and secondary B cells by cross-reacting determinants. J Exp Med 138: 1276–1281
Klinman NR, Press JL, Pickard AR, Woodland RT, Dewey AF (1974) Biography of the B cell. In: Sercarz E, Williamson A, Fox CF (eds) The immune system. Academic, New York, pp 357–365

Klinman NR, Pickard AR, Sigal NK, Gearhart PJ, Metcalf ES, Pierce SK (1976) Assessing B cell diversification by antigen receptor and precursor cell analysis. Ann Immunol 127: 489–502
Krawinkel U, Zoebelein G, Burggemann M, Radbruch M, Rajewsky K (1983) Recombination between antibody heavy chain variable-region genes: evidence for gene conversion. Proc Natl Acad Sci USA 80: 4997–5001
Linton P-J, Klinman, NR (1986) The generation of secondary B cells in vitro (abstract). Fed Proc 45: 378
Linton P-J, Gilmore GL, Klinman NR (1988) The secondary B cell lineage. In: Witte O, Howard M, Klinman NR (eds) B cell development. UCLA Symposia on Molecular and Cellular Biology, New Series, vol 85. Liss, New York
Linton PJ, Decker DJ, Klinman NR (1989) Primary antibody-forming cells and secondary B cells are generated from separate precursor cell subpopulations. Cell 59: 1049–1059
MacLennan ICM, Gray D (1986) Antigen-driven selection of virgin and memory B cells. Immunol Rev 91: 61–85
Makela O, Karjalainen K (1977) Inherited immunoglobulin idiotypes of the mouse. Immunol Rev 34: 119–138
Manser T (1987) Mitogen-driven B cell proliferation and differentiation are not accompanied by hypermutation of immunoglobulin variable region genes. J Immunol 139: 234–238
Manser T, Wysocki LJ, Margolies MN, Gefter ML (1987) Evolution of antibody variable region structure during the immune response. Immunol Rev 96: 141–162
McKean D, Huppi K, Bell M, Staudt L, Gerhard W, Weigert M (1984) Generation of antibody diversity in the immune response of BALB/c mice to influenza virus hemagglutinin. Proc Natl Acad Sci USA 81: 3180–3184
Metcalf ES, Klinman NR (1976) In vitro tolerance induction of neonatal murine B Cells. J Exp Med 143: 1327–1340
Metcalf ES, Klinman NR (1977) In vitro tolerance of bone marrow cells: a marker for B cell maturation. J Immunol 118: 2111–2116
Morrow PR, Jemmerson RRW, Klinman NR (1987) Disparities in the repertoire of B cells responsive to a native protein and those responsive to a synthetic peptide. In: Sercarz EE, Berzofsky J (eds) Immunogenicity of protein antigens: repertoire and regulation, vol II. Academic, Orlando, pp 43–49
Mosmann TR, Cherwinski H, Bond MW, Giedlin MA, Coffman RL (1986) Two types of murine helper T cell clones. I. Definition according to profiles of lymphokine activities and secreted proteins. J Immunol 136: 2348–2357
Nossal G, Warner N, Lewis H (1971) Incidence of cells simultaneously secreting IgM and IgG antibody to sheep erythrocytes. Cell Immunol 2: 41–53.
Nossal GJV, Pike BL (1975) Evidence for the clonal abortion theory of B lymphocyte tolerance. J Exp Med 141: 904–917
Owen FL, Nisonoff A (1978) Effect of idiotype-specific suppressor T cells on primary and secondary responses. J Exp Med 148: 182–194
Perlmutter RM, Crews ST, Douglas R, Sorensen G, Johnson N, Nivera N, Gearhart PJ, Hood L (1984) The generation of diversity in phosphorylcholine binding antibodies. Adv Immunol 35: 1–37
Pierce SK, Klinman NR (1977) Antibody-specific immunoregulation. J Exp Med 146: 509–519
Press JL, Klinman NR (1973) Monoclonal production of both IgM and IgG1 anti-hapten antibody. J Exp Med 135: 300–305
Raychaudhuri S, Cancro MP (1985) Cellular basis for neonatally induced T-suppressor activity. J Exp Med 161: 816–831
Riley RL, Klinman NR (1985) Differences in antibody repertoires for (4-hydroxy-3-nitrophenyl)acetyl (NP) in splenic vs immature bone marrow precursor cells. J Immunol 135: 3050–3055
Riley RL, Klinman NR (1986) The affinity threshold for antigenic triggering differs for tolerance susceptible immature precursors vs mature primary B cells. J Immunol 136: 3147–3154
Riley RL, Wylie DE, Klinman NR (1983) B cell repertoire diversification precedes immunoglobulin receptor expression. J Exp Med 158: 1733–1738
Selsing E, Storb U (1981) Somatic mutation of immunoglobulin light chain variable region genes. Cell 25: 47–58
Siekevitz M, Kocks C, Rajewsky K, Dildrop R (1987) Analysis of somatic mutation and class switching in naive and memory B cells generating adoptive primary and secondary responses. Cell 48; 757–770
Sigal NH, Klinman NR (1978) The B cell clonotype repertoire. Adv Immunol 26: 255–337

Stashenko P, Klinman NR (1980) Analysis of the primary anti-(4-hydroxy-3-nitrophenyl)acetyl (NP) responsive B cells in BALB/c and B10.D2 mice. J Immunol 125: 531–537
Stocker JW (1977) Tolerance induction in maturing B cells. Immunology 32: 282–290
Strober S (1972) Initiation of antibody responses by different classes of lymphocytes. V. Fundamental changes in the physiological characteristics of virgin thymus-independent ("B") lymphocytes and "B" memory cells. J Exp Med 136: 851–871
Symington FW, Hakemori S-I (1984) Hematopoietic subpopulations express cross-reactive, lineage-specific molecules detected by monoclonal antibody. Mol Immunol 21: 507–514
Teale JM, Klinman NR (1980) Tolerance as an active process. Nature 288: 385–386
Teale JM, Klinman NR (1984) Membrane and metabolic requirements for tolerance induction of neonatal B cells. J Immunol 133: 1811–1817
Teale JM, Lafrenz D, Klinman NR, Strober S (1981) Immunoglobulin class commitment exhibited by B lymphocytes separated according to surface isotype. J Immunol 126: 1952–1957
Wang A, Wilson A, Hopper J, Fudenberg H, Nisonoff A (1970) Evidence for control of synthesis of the variable regions of the heavy chains of immunoglobulins G and M by the same gene. Proc Natl Acad Sci USA 66: 337–343
Williamson AR, Zitron IM, McMichael AJ (1976) Clones of B lymphocytes: their natural selection and expansion. Fed Proc 35: 2195–2201
Yokota T, Arai N, de Vries JE, Spits H, Banchereau J, Zlotnick A, Rennick D, Howard M, Takebe Y, Miyatake S, Lee F, Arai K (1988) Molecular biology of interleukin 4 and interleukin 5 genes and biology of their products that stimulate B cells, T cells and hemopoietic cells. Immunol Rev 102: 137–187

# The Evolution of B-Cell Clones

I. C. M. MacLennan, Y. J. Liu, S. Oldfield, J. Zhang, and P. J. L. Lane



## 1 Introduction

Large numbers of B cells are produced throughout life as the result of both primary B lymphopoiesis (Opstelten and Osmond 1983) and antigen-driven B-cell proliferation (Fliedner et al. 1964). It is a feature of the system that a high proportion of the cells produced have a brief lifespan (Kumararatne et al. 1985; Freitas et al. 1986; MacLennan and Gray 1986). Some, however, survive for

Department of Immunology, The Medical School, University of Birmingham, Birmingham B15 2TJ, United Kingdom

Current Topics in Microbiology and Immunology, Vol. 159

much longer following positive selection. This can be antigen-dependent (MACLENNAN and GRAY 1986; GRAY et al. 1986). but may also be antigen-independent (MACLENNAN 1987). The B cells which migrate between the follicles of secondary lymphoid tissues and those which are located in the marginal zones of the spleen have been positively selected in this way. These cells, which are not in cell cycle, have an average lifespan of around 1 month (GRAY 1988a; GRAY and SKARVALL 1988). If they are not activated by antigen within this period they die.

Some B-cell clones, as opposed to individual B cells, have been shown to have an almost indefinite lifespan. These are the clones which maintain the established phase of T-cell-dependent antibody responses (GRAY et al. 1986). Such clones can dominate a specific antibody response throughout the lifespan of a rat or mouse and can be transferred to dominate the response to the same antigen in a syngeneic recipient (ASKONAS et al. 1970). It is probable that these clones are sustained by B blasts, which remain in antigen-driven cell cycle in the follicles of secondary lymphoid organs. This chapter will discuss antigen-dependent B-cell proliferation and selection in vivo and compare the relative contribution of memory and virgin B cells to these processes.

## 2 Virgin B-Cell Recruitment and Persistence of Memory B-Cell Clones in T-Cell-Dependent Antibody Responses

The use of chimaeras constructed between congenic strains of rats which differ in κ-immunoglobulin light chain allotype is discussed in detail in the chapter by DAVID GRAY and TOMAS LEANDERSON in this volume. These chimaeras have been particularly useful for analysing virgin B-cell recruitment and the persistence of memory B-cell clones in antibody responses. For this purpose chimaeras have been constructed so that primary B lymphopoietic capacity is confined to one allotype but most peripheral B cells are initially of the other allotype. This was originally achieved by exposing host rats to whole body irradiation with hind limb shielding and reconstituting these animals with thoracic duct lymphocytes from congenic donors. Using this system it was found that virgin B-cell recruitment in responses to the T-cell-dependent antigens was confined largely to those periods immediately following exposure to antigen. The established phase of the response was maintained by continued activation of memory B-cell clones, without further B-cell recruitment (GRAY et al. 1986).

Recently, similar results have been obtained following transfer of memory cells into non-irradiated rats which had not been previously immunized. In this case the donors were several months into the established phase of a secondary response to the T-cell-dependent antigen 2,4-dinitrophenyl ovalbumin (DNP-OA). Details of these experiments are shown in Fig. 1. In the first week after immunizing the chimaeras with DNP-OA, the anti-DNP response was mainly

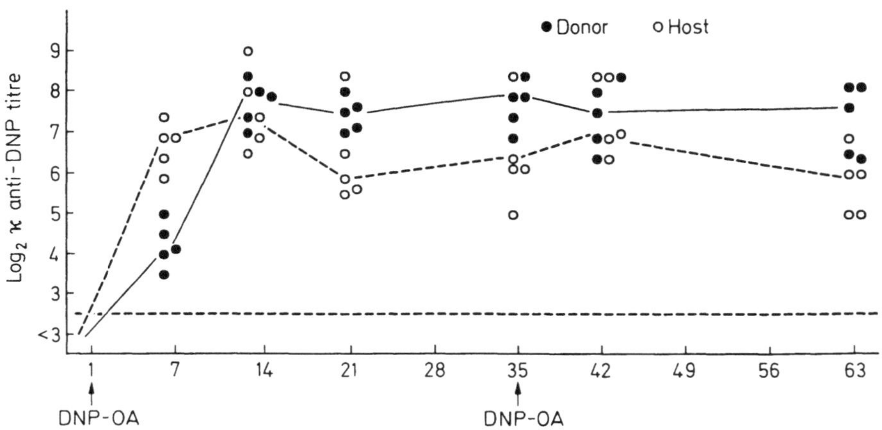


**Fig. 1.** Recruitment of virgin B cells and persistence of memory B-cell clones in responses to hapten-protein. Large numbers of virgin B lymphocytes are recruited into a response to a T-cell-dependent antigen in the period immediately following antigen administration. The established phase of the response is maintained by memory B-cell clones with little further virgin B-cell recruitment. Lymph node lymphocytes ($5 \times 10^7$) were transferred from PVG-κ-1a rats 6 months after they had received a secondary challenge with DNP-OA. The recipients were normal congenic PVG κ-1b rats which had not been previously immunized. The anti-DNP antibody responses of both donor (*solid line*) and host (*broken line*) origin after the chimaeras were challenged with soluble DNP-OA i.v. are shown. After one week the response was predominantly of host origin; suggesting that host DNP-reactive virgin B cells outnumbered the donor memory B cells and were well able to compete for activation by the antigen. Seven days later the donor anti-DNP antibody titres had reached comparable levels to those of the host and thereafter in all but one chimaera the donor cells dominated the response even after further challenge with DNP-OA. Details of the congenic strains of rats and the κ-allotype-specific anti-DNP assay are given in GRAY et al. (1986)

attributable to cells of host origin; suggesting that there were more DNP-reactive virgin B cells of host origin than donor memory B cells. At this stage, when free antigen was available, the virgin B cells were able to compete favourably with memory cells. Over the next week, however, donor clones progessively came to dominate the response and host anti-DNP antibody titres began to fall. By 3 weeks the relative proportions of anti-DNP antibody of donor and host origin which were to be maintained throughout the established phase of the response were reached. The donor dominance, which was established in the majority of chimaeras, does not seem to be due to suppression of the host allotype because (a) a significant level of host anti-DNP antibody production remained in all chimaeras in the established phase of the response and (b) when chimaeras showing donor dominance to DNP-protein are reimmunized with a combination of DNP-protein plus oxazolone (Ox) conjugated to the same protein, the anti-Ox response is almost exclusively of host allotype while the donor allotype continues to dominate the anti-DNP response. This second observation seems to exclude the possibility that donor dominance of the anti-DNP response resulted from bone marrow chimaerism being established. Secondary transfer experiments of bone marrow from chimaeras constructed with κ-allotype-marked lymph node cells or thoracic duct lymphocytes indicate that haemopoietic stem cells are not transferred in these primary donor populations (MACLENNAN and LOWE, unpublished data).

# 3 B-Cell Activation In Vivo in Responses to T-Cell-Dependent Antigens

## 3.1 Background

The series of experiments outlined in the previous section led to speculation that B cells might be activated in different sites at different stages in antibody responses. It was suggested that B-cell proliferation occurs in T-cell-rich areas in association with interdigitating cells (T zones) during periods immediately following antigen administration and that during the established phase of antibody responses this takes place in B-cell follicles, where a rich network of antigen-retaining follicular dendritic cells is located (MACLENNAN and GRAY 1986). Studies using techniques which allow antigen-specific B cells to be indentified in tissue sections (LIU et al. 1988) have indicated that this is the case. The level of complexity, however, is greater than was originally proposed, particularly in relation to the follicular response, which also has an important role shortly after antigen is given. B-cell activation in these two sites will be considered in some detail as they appear to provide the microenvironments in which memory B cells are generated. Follicles, in addition, by virtue of the antigen-retaining capacity of follicular dentritic cells (FDCs; TEW and MANDEL 1978, 1979), provide a site for positive selection of antigen-specific B cells. The mechanism of this selection and the fate of those cells which are not selected will be discussed in Sect. 6. It will be shown that memory cells generated through antigen-driven B-cell proliferation colonize the marginal zones of the spleen and to a lesser extent the follicular mantles (Sect. 5). The marginal zones, however, are not significant sites of antigen-driven B-cell proliferation; but if cells encounter antigen in these zones they can be induced to move to the sites of B-cell proliferation mentioned above.

## 3.2 Technical Considerations

Hapten-specific B cells can be identified using the haptens DNP or Ox conjugated to either alkaline phosphatase or horseradish peroxidase. In this way both Ox-binding and DNP-binding cells can be seen in the same section (Fig. 2a; LIU et al. 1988). These techniques have been combined with analysis of the proportion of cells in S phase of the cell cycle. For this purpose rats were injected with 5-bromo-2′-deoxyuridine (BrdUrd) 2 h before tissues were taken for

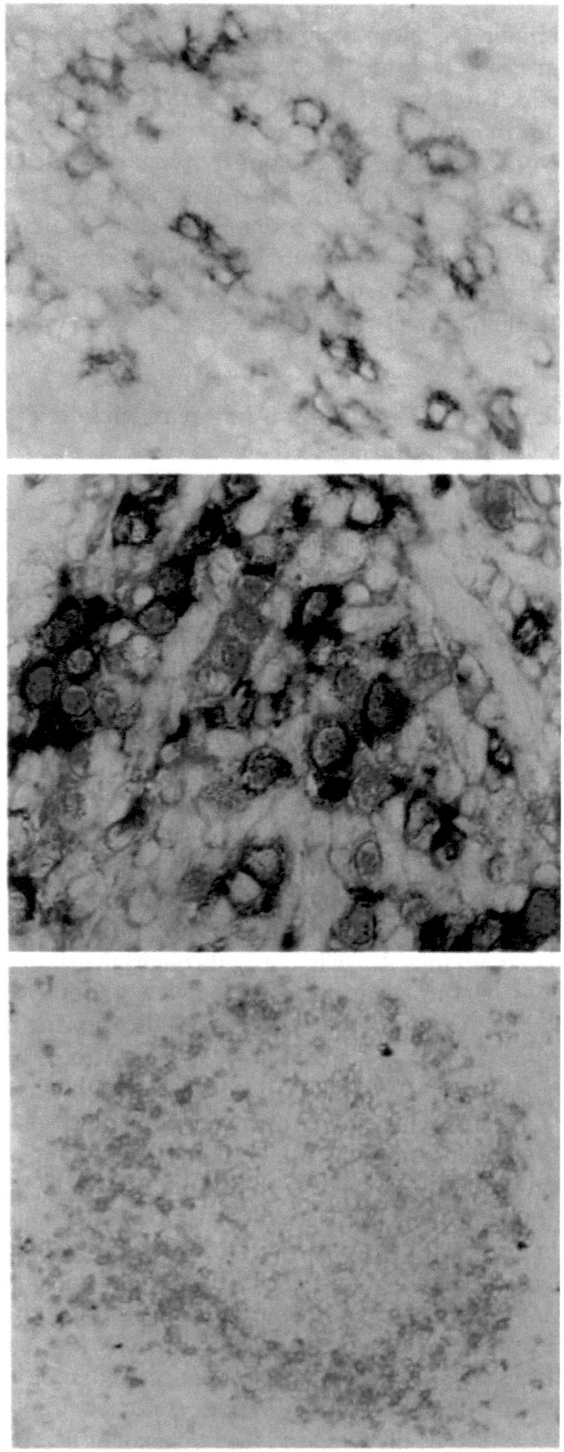

a b c

**Fig. 2. a.** Photomicrograph of an area of marginal zone from a rat spleen stained to identify Ox-binding B cells (*red*) and DNP-binding cells (*blue*). The rat had been primed with 50 $\mu$g alum-precipitated DNP-MSH with $10^9$ killed *Bordetella pertussis* organisms i.p. One month later it was boosted i.v. with 50 $\mu$g of soluble DNP-MSH and 50 $\mu$g soluble Ox-MSH. The spleen was removed and snap frozen for immunohistological examination 6 weeks later. Details of the staining technique are given in LIU et al. (1988). × 1000. **b** Photomicrograph of an area of T zone from a rat spleen stained to identify DNP-binding cells (*blue*), cells expressing the T-cell-associated antigen W3/13 (*gold*) and cells which had taken up BrdUrd into their nuclei in the 2 h before the spleen was removed for immunohistological examination (red). The rat was primed and boosted as described in **a** but was immunized for a third time with 50 $\mu$g soluble DNP-MSH 6 weeks after the second immunization. Massive accumulation of DNP-binding B blasts is seen in the T zones of this spleen, which was removed 36 h after the final challenge with DNP-MSH. Details of the staining technique are given in LIU et al. (1988). × 1000. **c** Photomicrograph of a rat spleen showing a secondary follicle. The follicular mantle cells are stained *gold* by indirect immunoperoxidase, which identifies HIS-22-binding cells. There are only very occasional HIS-22-binding cells in the follicle centre. × 150 immunohistological examination. Cells which had taken up this thymidine analogue were identified using an antibody specific for BrdUrd-containing DNA which has been treated with acid (CORDELL et al. 1984). The acid treatment destroys the activity of immunoenzymes previously applied to tissue sections without affecting the colour precipitate produced by these enzymes. Consequently, with a single section it is possible (a) to carry out double immunoenzyme staining, using a blue colour reaction with alkaline phosphatase and a yellow colour reaction with peroxidase and (b) after acid treatment, to reveal cells which have incorporated BrdUrd by red colour reaction. An example of this triple straining is shown in Fig. 2b.

### 3.3 B-Cell Proliferation in Areas Rich in T Cells and Interdigitating Cells

T zones are found in all secondary lymphoid organs, i.e. the spleen, lymph nodes, tonsils and mucosa-associated lymphoid tissues. They are the first sites at which hapten-specific B-cell proliferation is seen in response to hapten protein conjugates (MACLENNAN et al. 1988). Hapten-binding blasts are seen in these areas during the 2nd day after immunization provided that T help is not limiting, i.e. in carrier-primed animals or following secondary immunization with a hapten carrier. In these situations the B-cell proliferative response lasts only for about 48 h (Table 1), although in the first 3 days of a secondary response in the spleen the extent of extrafollicular proliferation can be impressive (Fig. 2b, Table 1). This response appears to be attributable to antigen-driven migration of memory B cells from the marginal zones into the T zones (Sect. 5.1; LIU et al. 1988). In primary B-cell responses, where there has been no priming with carrier and T help consequently is limiting, B-blast proliferation in T zones in very limited (Table 1).

B-blast reactions are most vigorous in the outer layers of T zones. Recirculating B cells pass through these areas on their way to follicles (NIEUWENHUIS and FORD 1976). Newly produced virgin B cells have also been shown to migrate into these areas after leaving the marrow. Few of these cells, however, pass on to the follicles unless they are positively recruited into the recirculating B-cell pool (LORTAN et al. 1987).

The T-cell-rich areas where these early B-blast reactions take place contain large numbers of interdigitating cells (sometimes termed dendritic cells). These cells are derived from haemopoietic stem cells in the bone marrow (FRELINGER et al. 1979; KATZ et al. 1979) and appear to be closely related to Langerhans' cells in the skin (SILBERGERG-SINAKIN et al. 1976; SCHULER and STEINMAN 1985). They express large amounts of class II MHC-encoded molecules (LAMPERT et al. 1980) and some macrophage-associated antigens (HOGG and HORTON 1987; MCKENZIE et al. 1987), but have little or no capacity for phagocytosis (FOSSUM et al. 1984). They also express the B-cell-associated molecules identified by CD40 and CDw78 monoclonal antibodies (LING et al. 1987). These interdigitating cells appear to be involved in T-cell-dependent B-cell activation (KNIGHT et al. 1982;

**Table 1.** The influence of T- and B-cell memory on the extent of the extrafollicular T-zone response to hapten-protein

| | Relative number[a] of DNP-binding B blasts in T zones at the peak of the extra-follicular response | | Days post-immunization of the peak of the extrafollicular B blast response | |
|---|---|---|---|---|
| | Median | Range | Day of peak | Start–end of response |
| Full primary response[b] | < 10 | < 10 | 6 | 4–7 |
| Primary B-cell response when T help not limiting[c] | 20 | 12–35 | 1.5 | 1.5–2.5 |
| Secondary B- and T-cell response[d] | 120 | 100–130 | 1.5 | 1–2.5 |

[a]The relative number of DNP-binding blasts is a value which is directly proportional to the number of these cells in the T zones of spleen (MACLENNAN et al. 1988)
[b]Immunization with 50 μg alum-precipitated DNP-MSH with $10^9$ killed *Bordetella pertussis* organisms i.p.
[c]Immunization with 50 μg soluble DNP-MSH and Ox-MSH i.v. 1 month after priming with 50 μg alum-precipitated MSH plus $10^9$ killed *Bordetella pertussis* organisms i.p.
[d]Immunization with 50 μg soluble DNP-MSH 6 weeks after priming and reimmunizing as in c

INABA et al. 1984). Although there is strong evidence that they are highly efficient at presenting antigen to T cells, it may also be that they provide an important microenvironment where B cells present antigen to T cells directly (MCKEAN et al. 1981; CHESNUT and GREY 1981; LANZAVECCHIA 1985). Possible explanations for these extrafollicular B-blast reactions being confined to the first few days following antigen administration include (a) the rapid turnover of interdigitating cells (FOSSUM et al. 1984) and (b) the possible inability of cells involved in this blast reaction to retain antigen for extended periods. Interdigitating cells differ markedly from FDCs in this respect. The extrafollicular responses seem likely to be of importance in

(a) recruiting virgin B cells into T-cell-dependent antibody responses and inducing them to progress to follicles (Sect. 5.2)
(b) initiating T-cell activation and inducing specific T-cell migration to follicles and
(c) generating short-lived plasma cells (see below).

The extrafollicular B-blast reaction is associated with the appearance of plasma cells in sites adjacent to those of B-cell activation. In the case of B-cell activation in the T zones of lymph nodes, the local sites of antibody secretion are the medullary cords of the same lymph node. In the spleen the corresponding site of antibody production is the red pulp. Plasma cells persist in these sites in substantial numbers for only 2–3 days after the extrafollicular B-blast reaction subsides. This is consistent with the finding that most antibody-producing cells in the spleen and lymph nodes of rats have a lifespan of less than 3 days (Ho et al. 1986). Continued antibody production after this initial period is by long-lived plasma cells whose precursors migrate to the bone marrow or lamina propria of the gut. The characteristics of plasma cells in these sites will be described in more detail in the next section.

## 3.4 Primary B-Cell Follicles

Follicular B-cell responses are complex, and a number of distinct phases in these responses can be recognized. This complexity is in part reflected in the diversity of the microenvironments in these structures which change markedly during the course of T-cell-dependent antibody responses. The structure of primary or resting follicles, i.e. those not supporting antigen-driven B-cell proliferation, is

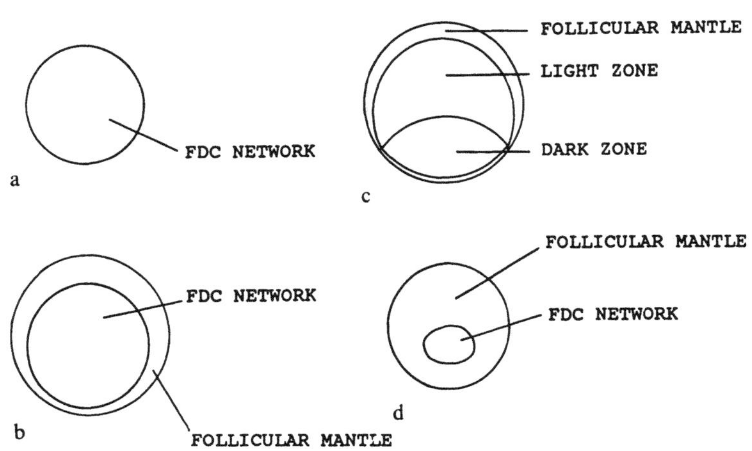


**Fig. 3a–d.** Phases of the follicular reaction during a T-cell-dependent antibody response from studies of rat spleen. **a** Primary follicle (pre-immunization). This consists of a single compartment with recirculating B cells filling the spaces in the *FDC network*. **b** Stage 1 secondary follicle (1–8 days after immunization). A few B blasts appear in the spaces of the *FDC network*. These proliferate and fill the space available. Recirculating B cells are displaced to form the *follicular mantle*. **c** Stage 2 secondary follicle (4–21 days after immunization). During this stage the *dark zone*, an area filled with centroblasts, forms. The FDC network fills with centrocytes and tingible bodies to form the *light zone*. Some B blasts remain. The time of onset of stage 2 depends upon whether T-cell help is limiting. When it is not, stage 2 starts at the end of the 4th day after immunization. This stage may not start until well into the 2nd week in fully primary responses. **d** Stage 3 secondary follicle (21 days to several months after immunization). The dark zone has involuted. Centrocytes are no longer present in the *FDC network* which has a *central core* of B blasts. Recirculating B cells of the *follicular mantle* enter the outer layer of the FDC network. (Further details are given in Table 2)

**Table 2.** Phenotypic differences between cells in secondary follicles

| a) B lineage cells | In cell cycle | sCD19 | sCD20 | sCD39 | sIgD | sIg | sCD38 | sCD10 |
|---|---|---|---|---|---|---|---|---|
| Recirculating follicular-mantle B cell | no | ++ | ++ | ++ | ++ | ++ | — | — |
| Follicular B blast | yes | ++ | ++ | — | — | ++ | ? | ? |
| Centroblast | yes | ++ | ++ | — | — | — | ++ | + |
| Centrocyte | no | ++ | ++ | — | — | + | ++ | + |

| b) FDC[a] | R4/23[b] | BU10[c] (2BF11) | CD21 (CR2) | CD23 | CD54 (ICAM-1) |
|---|---|---|---|---|---|
| Apical light zone | ++ | ++ | ++ | ++ | ± |
| Basal light zone | ++ | ++ | ++ | ± | ++ |
| Dark zone | ± | ± | ± | ± | ± |

| c) T cells | CD3 | CD4 | CD45Ro |
|---|---|---|---|
| Light zone only | ++ | ++ | ++ |

These phenotypic data are based upon analysis of secondary follicles in human tonsils
[a] IgA, IgM and IgG are taken up by FDC in association with antigen
[b] Stein et al. (1982)
[c] Johnson et al. (1986)

relatively simple (Fig. 3a). Their main cellular components are

(a) FDCs whose extensive dendritic processes form a dense central network which becomes progressively more dispersed towards the periphery of the follicle and
(b) recirculating surface (s)IgD$^+$ B cells, which fill the spaces in the FDC network.

The phenotype of FDCs and recirculating B cells is summarized in Table 2. In addition to these two major cellular elements of primary follicles there are small numbers of CD4$^+$ T cells (Stein et al. 1982), some macrophages and a capillary blood supply. In the splenic follicles there is a substantial minority of IgD$^-$ non-recirculating B cells, but these comprise fewer than 5% of follicular B cells in lymph nodes (Gray et al. 1982).

## 3.5 Secondary Follicle Formation

Secondary follicle formation is associated with antigen-driven B-cell proliferation, the germinal centre reaction, memory B-cell formation and plasma cell production. It can be divided into three distinct stages (MacLennan et al. 1988). Conventionally all three of these stages can be loosely considered under the term "germinal centre". We propose that this term be reserved for the second of the stages of secondary follicle formation described below:

**Stage 1.** B blasts appear in the FDC network. At this stage they are interspersed with small follicular B cells. The blasts proliferate rapidly until they become confluent, filling the follicle centre. The small recirculating B cells become displaced to the periphery of the follicle, forming the follicular mantle. The organization of cells associated with this stage of the follicular reaction is shown in Fig. 3b. A differential phenotype of cells involved in follicular reactions is given in Table 2.

**Stage 2.** This is the stage when the classical appearance of germinal centres develops. Shortly after B blasts become confluent in the follicle centre, phenotypically distinct blast cells (centroblasts) appear at one pole of the follicle (Fig. 3c). The area occupied by centroblasts is called the dark zone of a germinal centre and contains only a few terminal processes of FDCs. The dark zone in lymph nodes and splenic follicles is adjacent to the T zones. In Peyer's patches it is that part of the follicle nearest the peritoneum, and in tonsils it is the area furthest from the crypt epithelium. Centroblasts proliferate rapidly and are probably derived from the B blasts which developed in the first stage of follicular responses to antigen. At about the same time as the dark zone appears, the FDC network begins to fill with small irregularly shaped cells which are not in cell cycle. These are the progeny of centroblasts and are termed centrocytes. The area occupied by the centrocytes is known as the light zone of the germinal centre. It is the part of the follicle where the FDC network is thickest. At the peak of stage 2, centrocytes greatly outnumber the residual B blasts in the follicle centre. There is a high death rate amongst centrocytes and to a lesser extent centroblasts. The nuclear debris can be seen as intensely basophilic fragments (tingible bodies) within the macrophages of the germinal centre. The duration of the germinal centre reaction depends upon whether there is continued input of antigen. After a single injection of antigen, the germinal centre reaction is largely over within 3 weeks and the follicular reaction moves through to stage 3. The organization of human follicular cells during stage 2 of the follicular reaction is shown in Fig. 3c. The functional significance of germinal centres will be discussed in Sect. 6.

**Stage 3.** In this stage the light and dark zones are no longer apparent. Only a central core of B blasts remains. The size of this core is variable; the total volume is less than 10% of that seen at the height of a follicular reaction. This stage of the follicular response can continue for months and is probably maintained for the rest of the antibody response. The blast reaction appears to be driven by minute amounts of antigen which persist on FDCs (Tew and Mandel 1978, 1979). The organization of follicles during stage 3 of the follicular response is depicted in Fig. 3d.

## 3.6 Magnitude and Duration of Follicular Responses

The extent of proliferation during follicular responses varies considerably depending upon the level of pre-existing T-cell and B-cell memory and the availability of antigen. During chronic antigenic stimulation germinal centres are

**Table 3.** The influence of T- and B-cell memory on the extent of the follicular response to hapten-protein

| | Percentage splenic volume occupied by germinal centres at the height of the follicular response[a] | | Day after immunization of the peak of the follicular response |
|---|---|---|---|
| | Median | Range | |
| Fully primary response[b] | 0.4 | 0.2–1.0 | 10–14 |
| Primary B-cell response when T help not limiting[b] | 4.2 | 3.0–5.6 | 4 |
| Secondary B- and T-cell response[b] | 1.2 | 0.9–1.8 | 3 |

[a]The volume occupied by the follicular centre reaction was determined by counting the HIS22 negative area within follicles (Fig. 2c; KROESE et al. 1987a)
[b]Immunization procedures as described in Table 1. The results shown in this table are based upon analysis of the same rats as those which yielded the data given in Table 1

continuously present. This is apparent, for example, in human tonsils and Peyer's patches. Germinal centres, however, are frequently absent from normal human spleens and from the spleens of specific-pathogen free rodents. We have taken advantage of this negligible background of secondary follicles in the spleen to study the kinetics of germinal centre formation in rats. The size of germinal centres can be assessed accurately in rats using the monoclonal antibody HIS-22 (Fig. 2C; KROESE et al. 1987a). This stains follicular mantle B cells, but not germinal centre cells including follicular B blasts. Table 3 shows the volumes of the germinal centres in responses to hapten-protein conjugates. Availability of T-cell help appears to be the limiting factor determining the time of onset and extent of follicular proliferation in primary B-cell responses. This is seen by comparing the primary anti-hapten response following immunization with hapten-protein in carrier-primed rats with the response in previously non-immunized rats (Table 3). The hapten-binding blasts appear earlier and in far higher numbers in the carrier-primed rats. This effect does not appear to be due to the presence of anti-carrier antibody since passive transfer of antibody into previously non-immunized rats inhibits rather than promotes primary antibody responses when it is given at the time of immunization (KLAUS 1978; GRAY 1988b).

The volume of germinal centres in secondary responses to hapten-protein is only about a quarter of that associated with the response to hapten-protein in carrier-primed rats (Table 3). This finding suggests that cells which are virgin, rather than memory, at the time of antigen administration may be the principal or possibly exclusive contributors to stage 2 (the germinal centre stage) of the follicular reaction. This is consistent with the results obtained with $\kappa$-allotype congenic rats described in Fig. 1, i.e. virgin B cells can compete well with memory cells in the early phase of the response but memory cells tend to dominate the established phase. This will be considered further in Sect. 6.

### 3.7 Oligoclonal Nature of Follicular Responses

The oligoclonal nature of follicular responses was studied in the experiments described in Tables 1 and 3, where haemocyanin (MSH)-primed rats were challenged with Ox-MSH and DNP-MSH simultaneously. It was possible to determine the distribution of Ox-binding and DNP-binding cells within follicles in single sections as the follicular reaction developed. At the end of stage 1 of the follicular reaction, when the follicles were full of B blasts, most follicles contained variable mixtures of DNP-binding cells and Ox-binding cells. About 10% of the follicles, however, contained only Ox-binding or DNP-binding cells. One would expect to find single specificity follicles with such high frequency only if the average number of B blasts initiating the proliferative response in each follicle was low—certainly less than ten. KROESE et al. (1987b) studied the clonality of germinal centres following transfer of mixtures of congenic lymphocytes differing in CD45 allotype into lethally irradiated rats. They found an even higher proportion of follicles colonized by cells of a single allotype than the proportion of follicles we found containing B cells reacting with a single hapten. They concluded that follicular reactions were normally initiated by one or two B cells. The higher frequency of monoclonal follicles in their experiments may reflect a smaller number of antigen-reactive precursors being available in their chimaeras than in our non-irradiated rats. In any case both sets of experiments indicate that responses within individual follicles are oligoclonal.

## 4 Antibody Production Associated with Follicular Responses

It seems probable that the B blasts, which are present in all three stages of the follicular reaction, give rise to the plasma cells. Those associated with stage 3 are the most obvious precursors of the antibody-producing cells which maintain antibody production throughout the established phase of T-cell-dependent antibody responses. Characteristically, antibody production at this stage is distant from the site of B-cell activation. Plasmablasts are produced which migrate via the lymph and/or blood either (a) to the bone marrow, in the case of B-cell activation in the spleen or peripheral lymph nodes (BENNER et al. 1981); or (b) to the lamina propria of the gut, when B cells are activated in mesenteric lymph nodes or gut-associated lymphoid tissue (GOWANS and KNIGHT 1964; HALL et al. 1977). Bone marrow plasma cells producing IgG and IgA and about half the plasma cells of the lamina propria of the gut have a lifespan of the order of 1 month (HO et al. 1986). In this respect they differ markedly from the short-lived plasma cells of the spleen and lymph nodes, which are associated with the early days of T-cell-dependent antibody responses.

# 5 Memory B-Cell Production During T-Cell-Dependent Antibody Responses

The immunohistological techniques described earlier (Sect. 3.2) can be used to study the distribution of memory B cells. In this context a memory B cell is a cell which has undergone antigen-driven proliferation but is now no longer in cell cycle. During splenic responses to hapten-protein conjugates the most obvious sites of hapten-binding memory B-cell accumulation are the marginal zones (Fig. 2a). Relatively smaller numbers of hapten-binding cells are seen to accumulate in the follicular mantles.

## 5.1 Marginal Zone Memory B Cells

The marginal zones of the spleen form a major lymphoid compartment which is populated by phenotypically distinct B cells (KUMARARATNE et al. 1981; MACLENNAN et al. 1982). These cells express sIgM, but unlike recirculating follicular cells they have little or no sIgD (STEIN et al. 1980; GRAY et al. 1982). Substantial but variable minorities of these cells also express IgA or less commonly IgG (BAZIN et al. 1982). In man they display the B-cell-associated antigens recognized by CD19, CD20, CD21, CD22, CD37, CD39 and CD40 monoclonal antibodies (LING et al. 1987). They lack detectable CD23 antigen, and the leukocyte common antigen isotype recognized by the monoclonal antibody KiB3 (LING et al. 1987). Both of these antigens are associated with follicular mantle B cells. The marginal zones surround the follicles and in the rat, but not man, extend over the T-cell-rich areas of the white pulp. Unlike the follicles or T zones, which have a capillary blood supply, the marginal zones are perfused by a blood sinusoidal network which has its own direct arterial input. By this means the marginal zone B cells are particularly well placed to interact with antigens carried in the blood. There appear to be substantial numbers of cells similar to those found in the marginal zones beneath the dome epithelium of Peyer's patches (SPENCER et al. 1985). Small patches of these cells are also located on the inner wall of the subcapsular sinus of lymph nodes (STEIN et al. 1980; LIU et al. 1989). Both of these sites are well placed to allow direct contact between these cells and antigen.

Marginal zone cells do not appear to be derived directly from newly produced virgin B cells (LANE et al. 1986; LORTAN et al. 1987) but can develop from recirculating cells (KUMARARATNE and MACLENNAN 1981). There is evidence for antigen-independent entry of B cells in to the marginal zone, i.e. some transferred recirculating syngeneic B cells become marginal zone B cells without going through cell cycle in the recipient (OLDFIELD and MACLENNAN, unpublished observations). Techniques for detecting hapten-specific B cells in tissue sections have shown that memory B cells populate the marginal zones during T-cell-dependent antibody responses (LIU et al. 1988).

During simultaneous responses to Ox-protein and DNP-protein, discrete Ox-binding cells and DNP-binding cells colonize the marginal zones. This observations seems to exclude the possibility that cells in the marginal zone which bind hapten may do so because of passively bound antibody. Memory cells first appear in the marginal zones during stage 1 of the follicular response, before germinal centre formation and when B blasts are still active in T-cell-rich extrafollicular areas. There is no direct evidence to indicate whether marginal zone memory cells at this stage arise from both follicular and extrafollicular B blasts. In the established phase of T-cell-dependent antibody responses it seems probable that they are produced by stage 3 follicular blasts.

BrdUrd labelling studies indicate that marginal zone memory B cells are not, themselves, in cell cycle but that they are derived from proliferating precursors (Liu et al. 1988). This has been studied in rats primed with carrier protein during responses to hapten-protein. In these rats marginal zone hapten-binding cells reach near plateau levels 4 days after challenge with the hapten-protein. If the rats are given BrdUrd throughout the 3rd and 4th days of the response, a high proportion of marginal zone hapten-binding cells are found to be labelled. Analysis of the proportion of labelled hapten-binding cells at intervals after the BrdUrd pulse indicates that they have an average lifespan of a little under 3 weeks. About 40% of the labelled hapten-binding cells are found in the marginal zones 3 weeks after the BrdUrd pulse relative to the number present immediately after the pulse. These experiments were carried out in rats which had only been given a single intravenous injection of soluble antigen. Recent studies have shown that hapten-binding cells can still be found in the marginal zones 1 year after immunizing in this way. If the average lifespan of these cells is only 3 weeks, it follows that the production of marginal zone memory B cells continues throughout the established phase of T-cell-dependent antibody responses—presumably by B blasts. Production of marginal zone memory B cells must continue long after the germinal centre reaction (stage 2 of the follicular response) has ceased.

In the absence of further supplies of antigen, marginal zone memory cells appear to remain in this site until they die after about 3 weeks. If further antigen is injected, however, memory cells specific to that antigen are selectively induced to leave the marginal zones. This has been studied in rats in the established phase of a response to both Ox-protein and DNP-protein. If these animals are challenged with DNP-protein alone there is selective depletion of the DNP-binding cells of the marginal zone. Within the first few hours after this challenge there is a transient appearance of DNP-binding blasts in follicles. This transient migration to the follicles induced specifically by antigen is reminiscent of the non-specific mass migration of marginal zone B cells which is induced by injection of endotoxin (Petterson et al. 1967; Gray et al. 1984). It may be that these cells specifically transport antigen to FDCs. The role of marginal zone B cells in transporting antigen non-specifically in the form of immune complex has been subject to many studies (Brown et al. 1973; Gray et al. 1984; Kroese et al. 1986). The transient appearance of specific B blasts in the follicles is followed on the 2nd

**Table 4.** The ability of memory cells but not virgin cells, to respond to antigen localized in follicles

| Donor immunization | Antigen given with cells | κ-la anti-DNP response in recipient |
|---|---|---|
| 1. 1 month into a secondary response to MSH | None | Minimal |
| 2. 1 month into a secondary response to MSH | MSH | Minimal |
| 3. 1 month into a secondary response to MSH | DNP-MSH | Full |
| 4. 6 months into a secondary response to DNP-MSH | None | Full |
| 5. 6 months into a secondary response to DNP-MSH | DNP-MSH | Full |

*Experimental design.* Antigen was prelocalized on FDCs of PVG κ-lb rats by giving these rats DNP-MSH 1 month after priming them with MSH. Two days later they were irradiated with 600 cGy to destroy their lymphoid cells and 1 day after irradiation received congenic PVG κ-la spleen cells from animals immunized as indicated

*Comment.* The response in group 3 shows that antigen and the capacity for antigen presentation in follicles was not destroyed by irradiation. The failure of group 2 to respond indicates that the requirement for extrafollicular antigen is not to mobilize T help. The lack of requirement for extrafollicular antigen to obtain T-cell help is confirmed by the response obtained in group 4.

day after secondary challenge with DNP-protein by the massive T-zone blast reaction described in Sect. 3.3. It seems probable that memory cells derived from the marginal zones are the principal protagonists in this reaction.

Some 3 days after secondary challenge with DNP-protein, DNP-binding cells again colonize the marginal zones and rapidly reach the levels present before challenge. The delay before the return of these cells to the marginal zone (MacLennan et al. 1988) is considerably greater than that following endotoxin-induced migration of marginal zone cells to follicles (Gray et al. 1984). This suggests that the reappearance of specific memory cells in this site follows the generation of a fresh cohort of memory cells and not simply the return of the original cells.

## 5.2 Recirculating Virgin and Memory B Cells

Strober (1975) demonstrated that it was possible to transfer secondary antibody responses to irradiated syngeneic recipients with passaged thoracic duct lymphocytes. In these experiments, at best only poor responses were achieved in recipients of recirculating thoracic duct cells from non-immunized donors. Experiments described in detail by Gray and Leanderson in this volume and in Gray (1988b) provide evidence that congenic memory cells, but not virgin B cells, can respond to antigen localized in follicles on FDCs. We have obtained similar results using a different approach in experiments summarized in Table 4. If these results mean that only recirculating memory cells can respond to antigen already localized on FDCs, does it follow that the small B cells which recirculate between the follicles of secondary lymphoid organs are exclusively memory cells? There are a number of reasons for supposing that this may not be the case. This reasoning, however, makes it necessary to accept the paradox that although some virgin B cells do recirculate through follicles they can only become follicular B blasts if they encounter antigen outside follicles.

The following data would be difficult to explain if the hypothesis that the recirculating B-cell pool is composed entirely of memory cells were correct:

1. Rats treated from birth with anti-igM and anti-IgD antibodies have very few or no detectable B cells in their secondary lymphoid organs at 6 weeks of age. If suppression of B-cell development is then stopped by giving rat IgM and IgD, the appearance of $sIgD^+$ cells within follicles starts within 48 h and is largely complete 5 days after stopping suppression (BAZIN et al. 1985). The rate at which follicles fill in this situation is such that a high proportion of B cells generated in the marrow over this period must be colonizing the follicles. It is hard to envisage that all of these cells are being recruited to enter follicles following antigen-driven B-cell proliferation, B-blast formation and memory B-cell production, especially as repopulation of the follicles is advanced before IgM plasma cells first appear at day 4 after stopping suppression. Similar results have been obtained following peripheral B-cell depletion using whole body irradiation with conservation of haemopoietic capacity by shielding the hind limbs (LANE et al. 1986). These data do not exclude a proliferation-independent selection procedure based either upon antigen or anti-idiotype. Evidence that such a selection process operates during ontogeny has been provided by the elegant experiments of Kearney's group (VAKIL and KEARNEY 1986; VAKIL et al. 1986). It is not clear to what extent the recruitment of B cells to the mature peripheral B-cell pool in adults, which does not involve antigen-driven B-cell proliferation, occurs by these complex idiotypic networks. If they are the dominant selection force during repopulation of depleted peripheral B-cell pools, then a remarkably high proportion of newly produced virgin B cells are selected by this means.
2. Follicular and marginal zone B-cell numbers can only be fully restored, following depletion, by recruitment of newly produced virgin B cells. This conclusion has been reached using rats which were depleted both of peripheral B cells and primary B lymphopoietic capacity (OLDFIELD, LIU and MACLENNAN, unpublished observations). Rats were given 800 cGy whole body irradiation. These animals were protected with a small number of syngeneic bone marrow cells. Bone marrow cells transferred in this way do not enter productive B lymphopoiesis until the end of the 3rd week following transfer. The irradiated rats also received $10^7$ thoracic duct lymphocytes from $\kappa$-allotype congenic donors which were undergoing an established secondary immune response to DNP-MSH. The chimaeras produced good anti-DNP responses when challenged with DNP-MSH. However, 17 days after transfer there were still only very limited numbers of small follicular B cells and these

were of donor allotype. By 7 weeks after transfer the secondary lymphoid organs of the chimaeras had been fully repopulated, but more than 97% of the small follicular B cells were of host origin. Up to 20% of the antibody in the chimaeras at this stage, however, was of donor allotype. It is difficult to explain these results unless (a) the mechanisms which regulate the number of memory B cells which enter the recirculating and marginal zone pools are independent of those which regulate the total number of cells in those pools and (b) there is a major virgin B-cell component among the small B cells of follicles.

3. The follicles of congenitally athymic rats and mice fill with small $sIgD^+$ B cells in a relatively normal way during ontogeny. This implies that development of recirculating B cells in these animals does not depend on T-cell-dependent B-cell proliferation, germinal centre formation and memory B-cell production.

# 6 B-Cell Selection During Affinity Maturation of Antibody Responses

## 6.1 The Role of Somatic Mutation in Immunoglobulin Variable Region Genes

As T-cell-dependent antibody responses progress there is an increase in the average affinity of the antibodies produced. This is largely attributable to the selection of B-cell clones in which increased affinity has arisen as the result of somatic mutation in the immunoglobulin variable region genes (Tonegawa 1983). Analysis of the appearance of plasmablasts which have somatic mutations in their rearranged *V* region genes has been studied by making hybridomas at different stages following immunization (Berek and Milstein 1987; Cumano and Rajewsky 1985). Such studies have investigated antibody responses where the immunoglobulin gene *V* segment used is restricted. The response of BALB/c mice to Ox-chicken serum albumin has been extensively studied in this respect. One week into the primary immune response to this antigen, hybridomas generated were found to have immunoglobulin *V* regions with the same *V*-$\kappa$ and V-H segments. At this stage no base pair substitutions were found in the *V* region genes (Kaartinen et al. 1983). One week later, while the anti-Ox hybridomas still used the same *V* segments in their immunoglobulin *V* region genes these now had multiple base pair substitutions (Griffiths et al. 1984; Berek et al. 1985).

Two suggestions have been made concerning the stage of B-cell maturation where somatic mutation occurs in *V* region genes. One proposes that the process takes places during primary B lymphopoiesis at the time immunoglobulin genes rearrange (Wabl et al. 1987). The second suggests that this occurs during antigen-driven B-cell proliferation (MacLennan and Gray 1986). These two possibilities are not necessarily mutually exclusive. The experiments described at the start of this chapter (Fig. 1) were designed to investigate the stage in B-cell

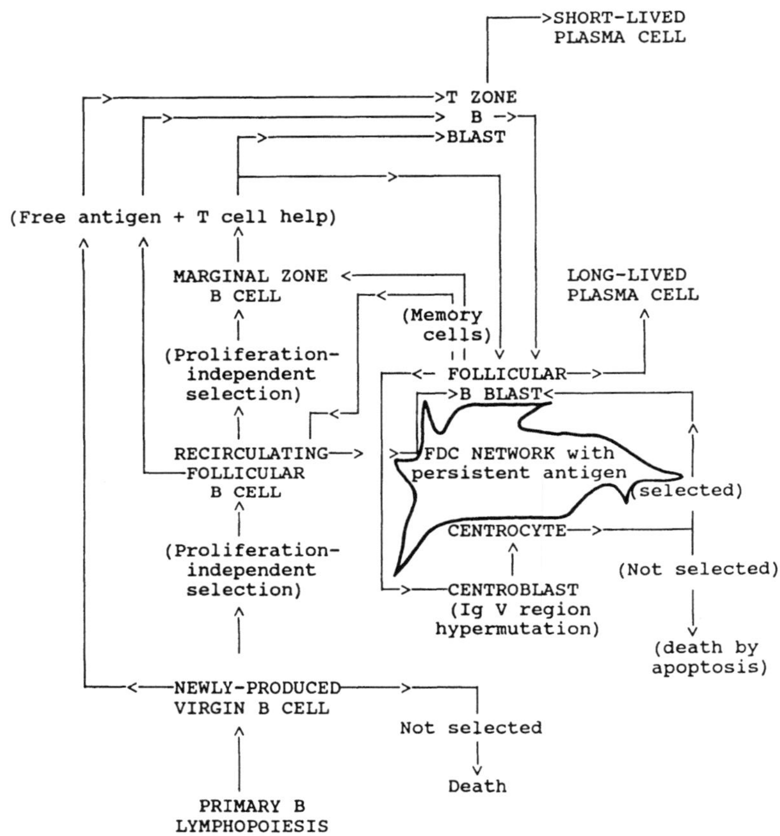


**Fig. 4.** Proposed pathways of B-cell differentiation in the rat based upon data cited in this chapter. Discussions of the various components of the diagram is set out in the following sections: Primary B lymphopoiesis and proliferation-independent recruitment of newly-produced virgin B cells into the recirculating pool of follicular B cells (Sects. 1, 5.2); recirculating follicular B cells (Sects. 3.4, 3.5, 5.2); marginal zone B cells and their origins (Sect. 5.1); T-zone B blasts (Sect. 3.3); FDCs (Sects. 2, 3.4–3.6, 5.1, 5.2, 6.1, 6.2); follicular B blasts (Sects. 2, 3.5–3.7, 5.2); centroblasts and centrocytes (Sects. 3.5, 3.6, 6.1, 6.2); somatic hypermutation (Sect. 6.1); selection of centrocytes in germinal centres (Sect. 6.2); short-lived plasma cells (Sect. 3.3); long-lived plasma cells (Sect. 4)

development at which somatic mutation occurs. These studies showed that virgin B-cell recruitment into responses to hapten-protein is largely confined to periods immediately following antigen administration. After this the response is maintained by repeated activation of memory B-cell clones. The findings apply equally to primary anti-hapten responses where carrier-primed lymphocytes are transferred and to adoptive secondary anti-hapten responses (Gray et al. 1986). The results of these experiments seem to favour the second proposal, namely that somatic mutation occurs principally during antigen-driven B-cell proliferation. If somatic hypermutation occurs at the time of primary immunoglobulin gene rearrangement, one would expect to see the emergence of clones derived from newly produced host virgin B cells during the 2nd and 3rd weeks of the response; however, by this stage the phase of virgin B-cell recruitment has already passed.

These experiments have led to the suggestion that a somatic hypermutation mechanism acting on immunoglobulin *V* region genes is selectively activated in centroblasts in the dark zone of germinal centres (MacLennan and Gray 1986). Siekevitz et al. (1987) looked for evidence of somatic mutation occurring in transferred memory B-cell clones. These clones had undergone extensive somatic mutation during the primary responses in the donor. It was found that the transferred B cells could go through extensive antigen-driven proliferation in the syngeneic recipient without further mutations arising in their immunoglobulin *V* regions. This finding is consistent with the suggestion put forward in Sect. 3.6 that virgin cells rather than memory cells are the precursors of centroblasts. Memory cells, however, will proliferate in response to antigen as B blasts either in the T zones (Sect. 3.3) or on the surface of FDCs (Sect. 3.5) No direct evidence has yet been obtained which identifies a hypermutation mechanism in centroblasts (Gray and Leanderson, this volume). Equally, we are not aware of data which make the proposal untenable. Figure 4 sets out the proposed sequence of cell maturation and selection in germinal centres.

## 6.2 Antigen-Driven Selection of B Cells Within Germinal Centres

Centroblast proliferation within the dark zone of germinal centres occurs with a cell cycle time of 7 h (Zhang et al. 1988a). Pulse labelling studies using tritiated thymidine (Fliedner et al. 1964) or BrdUrd (MacLennan et al. 1988) indicate that centrocytes, although not themselves in cell cycle, only stay for a matter of hours in the light zone. They are being continually replaced from the proliferating pool of centroblasts in the dark zone. Two fates for centrocytes have been identified: either they die within a few hours of entering the light zone or they give rise to memory B cells (Klaus et al. 1980; Coico et al. 1983). The death of centrocytes in the light zone is confirmed in the pulse labelling experiments cited above. Labelled nuclear debris is found within the macrophages of the light zone within 12 h of pulsing with thymidine or BrdUrd. It seems plausible that the high death rate in centrocytes reflects an active process of antigen-based selection. Evidence supporting this hypothesis which indicates how the mechanism of selection works has been produced by the analysis of cells isolated from the germinal centres of human tonsils (Liu et al. 1989).

Centroblasts and centrocytes in human tonsils have a characteristic phenotype which allows them to be separated from other tonsillar B-lineage cells (Ling et al. 1987; MacLennan et al. 1988; Fig. 3c). Of particular use in this respect has been their lack of both sCD39 antigen and sIgD and their failure to penetrate a 60% Percoll gradient. This allows them to be isolated to a high level of purity. Details of this separation procedure are set out in Table 5. Providing the separation is carried out at 4°C the viability of the isolated cells is good. If they are

**Table 5.** The high death rate in germinal centre B cells isolated from human tonsil and its prevention by activation with anti-immunoglobulin and CD40 antibody

| B-cell fraction | Additives to culture medium | Percentage of cells viable after culture at 37°C for: | |
|---|---|---|---|
| | | 16 h | 40 h |
| Heavy Small resting[b] | None | 96–99 | 60–81 |
| Medium + Light Germinal centre cell-depleted[c] | None | 87–95 | 68–90 |
| Germinal centre cell-enriched[d] | None | 26–14 | 0 |
| Germinal centre cell-enriched | Anti-Ig coated SRBC | 82–70 | 27–19 |
| Germinal centre cell-enriched | CD40 | 87–63 | 55–23 |
| Germinal centre cell-enriched | CD40 + anti-Ig coated SRBC | 92–80 | 82–68 |

[a] B cells were isolated from human tonsil cell suspensions by removing T cells by two cycles of rosetting with AET-modified sheep red blood cells (SRBC) and separating the rosetting cells on a Ficoll-Paque gradient.
[b] Cells of the B-cell fraction which penetrated a 60% Percoll gradient.
[c] Cells of the B-cell fraction not penetrating a 60% Percoll gradient which did not rosette with CD38-coated SRBC. CD38 is expressed by all germinal centre B-lineage cells but not by follicular mantle and most extrafollicular B cells.
[d] Cells of the B-cell fraction not penetrating a 60% Percoll gradient which did not rosette with either IgD-coated or CD39-coated SRBC.

cultured at 37°C, however, they rapidly undergo self-destruction by apoptosis, so that on average only 10%–20% of the starting population is viable after a 16h culture. The occurrence of apoptosis in these cells has been confirmed on morphological grounds both at the electron and light microscopic levels as well as by identification of the DNA fragmentation pattern which characterizes this process (WYLLIE et al. 1984; SMITH et al. 1989). Culture of other medium-to-low density B cells which lack the phenotypic features of germinal centre cells is not associated with significant apoptosis during 48-h culture. This equally applies to dense follicular mantle-cell-rich tonsillar B cells.

The high death rate of cultured germinal centre cells seems to reflect the equally impressive rate of cell death which is observed in these cells in vivo (FLIEDNER et al. 1964). Further experiments have shown that these cells can be prevented from entering apoptosis if they are activated through their surface receptors for antigen (Table 2). This is achieved by culturing the isolated germinal centre cells with anti-human immunoglobulin which has been conjugated to sheep red cells. (Soluble anti-immunoglobulin is ineffective in this respect.) It has not been possible to rescue these cells by a range of soluble B-cell growth and activation factors used singly or in combination, i.e. a trigger via the antigen-specific receptor of the centrocyte seems to be required for rescue. Recently it has become apparent that the CD40 antibody G28-5 also has the capacity to prevent apoptosis. The inclusion of this as well as anti-immunoglobulin on sheep red cells achieves a more complete prevention of apoptosis in germinal centre cells than either agent applied alone (Table 5). The natural ligand for the antigen recognized by CD40 antibodies is unknown, although this molecule has homology with nerve growth factor receptor. It is tempting to speculate that the rescue signal for centrocytes delivered through this molecule is provided in vivo by interaction with FDCs.

Phenotypic analysis of the tonsil germinal fraction shows that only about 60% of these cells express surface immunoglobulin and this is almost exclusively IgG. This is consistent with the observation that centroblasts in vivo express little or no surface immunoglobulin but that when they come out of cell cycle and move to the light zone as centrocytes they re-express it. In the germinal centres in Peyer's patches the immunoglobulin isotype expressed by centrocytes is mainly IgA (Butcher et al. 1982).

# 7 T-Cell-Independent B-Cell Activation

Many of the experimental procedures applied to the analysis of T-cell-dependent (TD) B-cell activation in the rat have been applied to the study of T-cell-independent (TI) B-cell activation.

## 7.1 TI-2 Antigens

Responses to haptenated polysaccharides such as Ficoll and hydroxyethyl starch are strikingly different from responses to TD antigens. The polysaccharide-based antigens with one or two exceptions behave as TI-2 antigens (Mosier and Subbarao 1982), i.e. they fail to evoke antibody responses until late in development in normal individuals and do not normally give rise to antibody production in CBA/N mice. Analysis of virgin B-cell recruitment and the persistence of memory B-cell clones in response to these antigens was assessed using the experimental system described in Sect. 2. These experiments indicated that there is continued recruitment of virgin B cells during these responses and that activated B-cell clones at best only persist for a few weeks (Lane et al. 1986). Although virgin B cells are recruited into these responses, it appears that neither newly produced virgin B cells nor recirculating B cells are activated by these antigens. They appear only to be able to evoke a response from antigen-specific B cells which have colonized the marginal zones of the spleen and possibly equivalent cells in other lymphoid organs (Lane et al. 1986). The finding of Humphrey and Grennan (1981) that neutral polysaccharides localize to specialized dendritic cells located in the marginal zones may indicate a means by which continued recruitment of marginal zone B cells is achieved. Hapten-specific memory B cells do not colonize the marginal zones during responses to hapten-polysaccharide antigens (LIU et al. 1988). However, if bacterial lipopolysaccharide (LPS) is injected after rats have been immunized with hapten-polysaccharide, hapten-specific B cells do appear in the marginal zones (ZHANG et al. 1988b). Such synergy does not occur between TD and TI-2 antigens in rats.

### 7.2 TI-1 Antigens

Responses to the TI-1 antigen trinitrophenyl-LPS (TNP-LPS) in rats show a virgin B-cell recruitment pattern similar to that found in responses to TD antigens (ZHANG et al. 1988b). There is also persistent activation of memory B-cell clones in responses to TNP-LPS. Donor responses in chimaeras constructed between congenic strains of rat differing in $\kappa$-light chain allotype, as described in Sect. 2, can be detected for many months in responses to TNP-LPS. It has not been determined whether this persistence of the response is associated with T-cell activation by this antigen.

TI-1 antigens do induce memory B cells which colonize the marginal zones of the spleen. This appears to be a TI process, for TNP-LPS will induce the formation of TNP-specific marginal zone memory B cells in nude rats. DNP-MSH induces marginal zone memory cells in nude rats. (LANE, unpublished observation) despite the failure of this antigen to evoke any antibody response in these animals (GRAY et al. 1985). Memory B-cell production without induction of antibody synthesis by TD antigens in nude mice has been described previously (SCHRADER 1975).

## 8 Summary and Conclusions

This chapter identifies three forms of B-cell memory: (a) B blasts which characterize the established stage of the follicular response to TD antigens, (b) recirculating memory B cells, and (c) non-recirculating memory B cells of the marginal zones of the spleen and equivalent areas of other secondary lymphoid organs. The follicular B blasts show sustained proliferation driven by small amounts of antigen bound to FDCs. The probable relationships between these cells is summarized diagrammatically in Fig. 4.

It is probable that follicular B blasts generate both the recirculating and marginal zone memory cells. The chapter by GRAY and LEANDERSON in this volume cites data which indicate that the recirculating memory pool is not sustained for more than a few weeks in the absence of antigen. Data leading to the same conclusion for marginal zone memory B cells is set out in Sect. 5.1 of this chapter. Marginal zone memory B cells do not appear to move spontaneously to follicles for periodic renewal. They will only leave the marginal zone if a fresh supply of antigen reaches them in that site. Recirculating B cells are able to respond to antigen already held on FDCs (Table 4). It is not known if they are able to displace B blasts of equivalent affinity for antigen which already occupy antigen-holding sites on FDCs. This could be a mechanism by which B blasts with high antigen affinity produced in one follicle could displace blasts of lower affinity in other follicles.

Little is known of the factors which regulate the numbers of marginal zone and recirculating follicular memory B cells. In responses to hapten-protein conjugates, hapten-binding cells may approach 10% of marginal zone B cells but comprise well under 1% of recirculating follicular cells. The numbers of these memory cells do not increase if the recirculating pool of lymphocytes is depleted, indicating that the factors which regulate the number of memory B cells are independent of those which regulate the total size of the recirculating B-cell pool. A depleted peripheral B-cell pool can only be fully reconstituted by recruitment of newly produced virgin B cells. Data cited in Sect. 5.2 support the concept that this recruitment is at least partially independent of antigen-driven B-cell proliferation. Consequently, substantial proportions of the peripheral B-cell pools are likely to be either virgin cells or cells which have been recruited by antigen or anti-idiotype without entering cell cycle.

During the first 2–3 weeks following exposure to TD antigen there is massive expansion of B-cell clones within follicles. The proliferative response in each follicle is oligoclonal. The high rate of cell division in follicles is matched by an equally impressive death rate among the B cells generated. Evidence is set out to indicate that this represents an ordered process of selection based on the survival of cells which can be activated by limited supplies of antigen on FDCs. Cells which do not receive this signal within a few hours destroy themselves by apoptosis. This selection process which characterizes the germinal centre stage of the follicular reaction is discussed in detail in Sects. 3.5, 3.6 and 6. It is suggested, on the basis of indirect evidence, that centroblasts within germinal centres activate a process which results in hypermutation within their rearranged immunoglobulin *V* region genes.

Extrafollicular B-cell activation appears to be confined to periods immediately following exposure to antigen. The significance of this to the rapid onset of antibody production and the recruitment of both T and B cells into antibody responses is considered in Sect. 3.3.

Finally, B-cell activation by TD and TI antigens is compared. Responses to antigens based on pure polysaccharide TI-2 antigens generate little or no memory B cells. They are only able to sustain B blasts in cycle for about 1 month. Responses to these antigens are sustained by continued virgin B-cell recruitment. Evidence is discussed which indicates that TI-2 antigens are only able to activate B cells which have colonized the marginal zones and equivalent areas. Antigens based upon LPS show B-cell recruitment patterns and memory cell formation which is much more closely related to that seen during TD responses.

*Acknowledgements.* The authors would like to thank Drs. MARIE KOSCO, GERALD JOHNSON and DAVID GRAY for reading the manuscript and making many helpful suggestions and the Medical Research Council for providing programme grant support for much of the work described in this chapter.

## References

Askonas BA, Williamson AR, Wright BG (1970) Selection of a single antibody-forming clone and its propagation in syngeneic mice. Proc Natl Acad Sci 67: 1398

Bazin H, Gray D, Platteu B, MacLennan ICM (1982) Distinct sIgD +vea and sIgD −ve B lymphocyte lineages in the rat. Ann NY Acad Sci 399: 157

Bazin H, Platteau B, MacLennan ICM, Johnson GD (1985) B-cell production and differentiation in adult rats. Immunology 54: 79

Benner R, Hijmans W, Haaijman JJ (1981) The bone marrow: the major source of immunoglobulins, but still a neglected site of antibody formation. Clin Exp Immunol 46: 1

Berek C, Milstein C (1987) Mutation drift and repertoire shift in maturation of the immune response. Immunol Rev 96: 23

Berek C, Griffiths GM, Milstein C (1985) Molecular events during maturation of the immune response to oxazalone. Nature 316: 412

Brown JC, Harris G, Papamichail M, Slijivic VS, Holborow EJ (1973) Localization of aggregated human gamma-globulin in the spleens of normal mice. Immunology 24: 955

Butcher EC, Rouse RV, Coffman RL, Nottenburg CN, Hardy RR, Weissman IL (1982) Surface phenotype of Peyer's patch germinal centre cells: implications for the role of germinal centers in B cell differentiation. J Immunol 129: 2698

Chesnut RH, Grey HM (1981) Studies of the capacity of B cells to serve as antigen presenting cells. J Immunol 126: 1075

Coico RF, Bhogal BS, Thorbecke GJ (1983) The relationship of germinal centres in lymphoid tissues to immunologic memory. VI. Transfer of B cell memory with lymph node cells fractionated according to their receptors for peanut agglutinin. J Immunol 131: 2254

Cordell JL, Falini B, Erber WW et al. (1984) Immunoenzymatic labeling of monoclonal antibodies using immune complexes of alkaline phosphates and monoclonal anti-alkaline phosphatase. J Histochem Cytochem 32: 219

Cumano A, Rajewsky K (1985) Structure of primary anti-(4-hydroxy-3-nitrophenyl) acetyl (NP) antibodies in normal and idiotypically suppressed C57BL/6 mice. Eur J Immunol 15: 512

Fliedner TM, Kress M, Cronkite EP, Robertson JS (1964) Cell proliferation in germinal centers of the rat spleen. Ann NY Acad Sci 113: 578

Fossum S, Rolsted N, Ford WL (1984) Thymus independence, kinetics and phagocytic ability of interdigitating cells. Immunobiology 168: 403

Freitas AA, Rochas B, Coutinho AA (1986) Lymphocyte population kinetics in the mouse. Immunol Rev 91: 5

Frelinger JG, Hood L, Hill S, Frelinger LA (1979) Mouse epidermal Ia molecules have a bone marrow origin. Nature 282: 321

Gowans JL, Knight EJ (1964) The route of recirculation of lymphocytes in the rat. Proc R Soc (Lond) B 159: 257

Gray D (1988a) Population kinetics of rat peripheral B cells. J Exp Med 167: 805

Gray D (1988b) Recruitment of virgin B cells into an immune response is restricted to activation outside lymphoid follicles. Immunology 65: 73

Gray D, Skarvall H (1988) B cell memory is short-lived in the absence of antigen. Nature 336: 70

Gray D, MacLennan ICM, Bazin H, Khan M (1982) Migrant $sIgM^+sIgD^+$ and static $sIgM^+$ $sIgD^-$ B lymphocyte subsets. Eur J Immunol 12: 564

Gray D, Kumararatne DS, Lorton J, Khan M, MacLennan ICM (1984) Relation of intra-splenic migration of marginal zone B cells to antigen localization on follicular dendritic cells. Immunology 52: 659

Gray D, Chassoux D, MacLennan ICM, Bazin H (1985) Selective depression of thymus-independent anti-DNP antibody responses induced by adult but not neonatal splenectomy. Clin Exp Immunol 60: 78

Gray D, MacLennan ICM, Lane PJL (1986) Virign B cell recruitment and the lifespan of memory during antibody responses to DNP-hemocyanin. Eur J Immunol 16: 641

Griffiths GM, Berek C, Kaartinen M, Milstein C (1984) Somatic mutation and the maturation of the immune response to 2-phenyloxazalone. Nature 315: 271

Hall JG, Hopkins J, Orlans E (1977) Studies on lymphoblasts in the sheep III: the destination of lymph-borne immunoblasts according to their tissue origin. Eur J Immunol 7: 30

Ho F, Lortan J, Kahn M, MacLennan ICM (1986) Distinct short-lived and long-lived antibody-producing cell populations. Eur J Immunol 16: 1297

Hogg N, Horton MA (1987) Myeloid antigens: new and previously defined clusters. In: McMichael et al. (eds) Leucocyte typing III. Oxford University Press, Oxford, p 576

Humphrey JH, Grennan D (1981) Different macrophage populations distinguished by means of fluorescent polysaccharides. Recognition and properties of marginal zone macrophages. Eur J Immunol 11: 221

Inaba K, Whitmer MD, Steinman RM (1984) Clustering of dendritic cells, helper T lymphocytes, and histocompatible B cells during primary antibody responses in vitro. J Exp Med 160: 858

Johnson GD, Hardie DL, Ling NR, MacLennan (1986) Human follicular dendritic cells: a study with monoclonal antibodies. Clin Exp Immunol 64: 205

Kaartinen M, Griffiths GM, Markham AF, Milstein C (1983) mRNA sequences define an unusually restricted IgG response to 2-phenyloxazalone and its early diversification. Nature 304: 320

Katz SI, Kunihiko T, Sachs DH (1979) Epidermal Langerhans' cells are derived from cells originating in the bone marrow. Nature 282: 324

Klaus GGB (1978) The generation of memory cells. II. Generation of B memory cells with performed antigen antibody complexes. Immunology 34: 643

Klaus GGB, Humphrey JH, Kunkle A, Dongworth DW (1980) The follicular dendritic cell: its role in antigen presentation in the generation of immunological memory. Immunol Rev 53: 3

Knight SC, Balfour BM, O'Brien J, Buttifant L, Sumersk T, Clarke J (1982) Role of veiled cells in lymphocyte activation. Eur J Immunol 12: 1057

Kroese FGM, Wabbena AS, Nieuwenhuis P (1986) Germinal centre formation and follicular antigen trapping in the spleen of lethally X-irradiated and reconstituted rats. Immunology 57: 99

Kroese FGM, Wabbena AS, Opstelten D et al. (1987a) B lymphocyte differentiation in the rat: production and characterization of monoclonal antibodies to B lineage-associated antigens. Eur J Immunol 17: 921

Kroese FGM, Wabbena AS, Seijen HG, Nieuwenhuis P (1987b) Germinal centers develop oligoclonally. Eur J Immunol 17: 1069

Kumararatne DS, MacLennan ICM (1981) Cells of the marginal zone of the spleen are derived from recirculating precursors. Eur J Immunol 11: 865

Kumararatne DS, Bazin H, MacLennan ICM (1981) Marginal zones: the major B cell compartment in rat spleens. Eur J Immunol 11: 858

Kumararatne DS, Gray D, MacLennan ICM, Lorton J, Platteau B, Bazin (1985) The paradox of high rates of B cell production in the bone marrow and the longevity of most mature B cells. Adv Exp Med Biol 186: 73

Lampert IA, Pizzola G, Thomas JA, Janossy GA (1980) Immunohistochemical characterization of cells involved in dermatopathic lymphadenopathy. J Pathol 113: 145

Lane PJL, Gray D, MacLennan ICM (1986) Differences in recruitment of virgin B cells into antibody responses to thymus-dependent and thymus-independent type-2 antigens. Eur J Immunol 16: 1569

Lanzavecchia A (1985) Antigen-specific interaction between T and B cells. Nature 314: 537

Ling NR, MacLennan ICM, Mason DY (1987) B cell and plasma cell antigens: new and previously defined clusters. In: McMichael et al. (eds) Leukocyte typing III. Oxford University Press, Oxford, pp 302–335

Lui Y-J, Joshna DE, Williams GT, Smith CA, Gordon J, MacLennan ICM (1989) Mechanism of antigen-driven selection in germinal centres Nature 342: 929

Liu Y-J, Oldfield S, MacLennan ICM (1988) Memory B cells in T cell-dependent antibody responses colonize the splenic marginal zones. Eur J Immunol 18: 355
Liu Y-J, Oldfield S, MacLennan ICM (1989) Thymus-independent type 2 responses in lymph nodes. Adv Exp Biol Med 237: 113
Lortan JE, Roobottom CA, Oldfield A, MacLennan ICM (1987) Newly-produced virgin B cells migrate to secondary lymphoid organs but their capacity to enter follicles is restricted. Eur J Immunol 17: 1311
MacLennan ICM (1987) In: Melchers F, Potter M (eds) Mechanisms in B cell neoplasia Roche, Basel, pp 63–73
MacLennan ICM, Gray D (1986) Antigen-driven selection of virgin and memory B cells. Immunol Rev 91: 61
MacLennan ICM, Gray D, Kumararatne DS, Bazin H (1982) The lymphocytes of the marginal zone: a distinct B lineage. Immunol Today 3: 305
MacLennan ICM, Liu Y-J, Ling NR (1988) B cell proliferation in follicles, germinal centre formation and the site of neoplastic transformation in Burkitt's Lymphoma. Curr Top Microbiol Immunol 141: 138
McKean DJ, Infante AJ, Nilson A, Kimoto M, Fanthman CG, Walker E, Warner N (1981) Major histocompatibility complex restricted antigen presentation to antigen-reactive T cells by B lymphocyte tumor cells. J Exp Med 154: 1419
McKenzie JL, Reid GF, Beard MEJ, Hart DNJ (1987) Reactivity of myeloid monoclonal antibodies with human dendritic cells. In: McMichael et al. (eds) Leukocyte typing III. Oxford University Press, Oxford, p 668
Mosier DE, Subbarao B (1982) Thymus-independent antigens: complexity of B lymphocyte activation revealed. Immunol Today 3: 217
Nieuwenhuis P, Ford WL (1986) Comparative migration of T and B cells in the rat spleen and lymph nodes. Cell Immunol 23: 254
Opstelten D, Osmond DG (1983) Pre-B cells in mouse bone marrow: immunofluorescence stathmokinetic studies of the proliferation of cytoplasmic u-chain-bearing cells in normal mice. J Immunol 131: 2635
Petterson JC, Borgen DF, Graupner KC (1967) A morphological and histochemical study of primary and secondary immune responses in rat spleen. Am J Anat 121: 305
Schrader JS (1975) The role of T cells in IgG production; thymus-dependent antigens induce B cell memory in the absence of T cells. J Immunol 114: 1665
Schuler G, Steinman RM (1985) Murine epidermal cells mature into potent immunostimulatory dendritic cells in vitro. J Exp Med 161: 526
Siekevitz M, Kocks C, Rajewsky K, Dildrop R (1987) Analysis of somatic mutation and class switching in naive and memory B cells generating adoptive primary and secondary responses. Cell 48: 578
Silberberg-Sinakin I, Thorbecke GJ, Baer RL, Rosenthal SA, Berezowsky V (1976) Antigen-bearing Langerhans' cells in skin, dermal lymphatics and in lymph nodes. Cell Immunol 25: 137
Smith CA, Williams GT, Kingston R, Jenkinson EJ, Owen JJT (1989) Antibodies to the CD3/T cell-receptor complex induce apoptosis (controlled cell death) in immature T cells in thymic cultures. Nature 337: 181
Spencer J, Finn T, Pulford KAF, Mason DY, Isaacson PG (1985) The human gut contains a novel population of B lymphocytes which resemble marginal zone cells. Clin Exp Immunol 62: 607
Stein H, Bonk A, Tolksdorf G, Lennart K, Rodt H, Gerdes J (1980) Immunohistologic analysis of the organization of normal lymphoid tissue and non-Hodgkin's lymphomas. J Histochem Cytochem 28: 746
Stein H, Gerdes J, Mason DY (1982) The normal and malignant germinal centre. Clin Haematol 11: 531
Strober S (1975) Immune function, cell surface characteristics and maturation of B cell subpopulations. Transplant Rev 24: 84
Tew JG, Mandel TE (1978) The maintenance and regulation of serum antibody levels: evidence indicating a role for antigen retained in lymphoid follicles. J Immunol 120: 1063
Tew JG, Mandel TE (1979) Prolonged antigen half-life in the lymphoid follicles of specifically immunized mice. Immunology 37: 69
Tonegawa S (1983) Somatic generation of antibody diversity. Nature 302: 575
Vakil M, Kearney JF (1986) Functional characterisation of monoclonal anti-idiotype antibodies isolated from the early B cell repertoire of BALB/c mice. Eur J Immunol 16: 1151

Vakil M, Sauter H, Paige, C, Kearney JF (1986) In vivo suppression of perinatal multispecific B cells results in distortion of the adult B cell repertoire. Eur J Immunol 16: 1159
Wabl M, Jäck HM, Meyer J, Beck-Engeser G, von Borstel RC, Steinberg CM (1987) Measurement of mutation rates in B lymphocytes. Immunol Rev 96: 91
Wyllie AH, Morris RG, Smith AL, Dunlop D (1984) Chromatin cleavage in apoptosis: association with condensed chromatin morphology and dependence on macromolecular synthesis. J Pathol 142: 67
Zhang J, MacLennan ICM, Liu Y-J, Lane PJL (1988a) Is rapid proliferation in B centroblasts linked to somatic mutation in memory B cell clones? Immunol Lett 18: 297
Zhang J, Liu Y-J, MacLennan ICM, Gray D, Lane PJL (1988b) B cell memory to thymus-independent type 1 and type 2: the role of lipopolysaccharide in B memory induction. Eur J Immunol 18: 1417

# Antiviral T-Cell Memory?

R. M. Zinkernagel



## 1 Introduction

Generally, it is accepted that immunological memory exists at both the B- and the T-cell level (reviewed in Katz 1977). It has been known for more than 100 years that the persistence of high antibody titers (Fig. 1) can be lifelong after viral infections and that delayed-type hypersensitivity can be demonstrated for a long time by challenging with a protein antigen after prior infection with tubercle bacilli. The concept of providing protection from disease by vaccination depends entirely on the existence of immunological memory. Although evidence for B-cell memory is abundant (Katz 1977), it is not clear whether it is maintained by means of (a) persistence of antigen, (b) continuous exposure to cross-reactive "natural" environmental antigen, or (c) the existence of true memory B cells.

The formal demonstration of T-cell memory has occurred more recently, and evidence for it has been summarized in various reviews (Katz 1977). The classic experiments showing T-cell memory involve carrier-specific T cells helping hapten-specific B cells. In many of these experiments T-cell memory was induced with persisting antigens because these antigens were injected along with adjuvants. Also, in these experiments, T-cell memory was often studied at a rather early stage, i.e., 3–8 weeks after priming, and usually hapten carrier responses

Institute of Pathology, University Hospital, CH-8091 Zürich, Switzerland
This review was submitted on 4 July 1988.

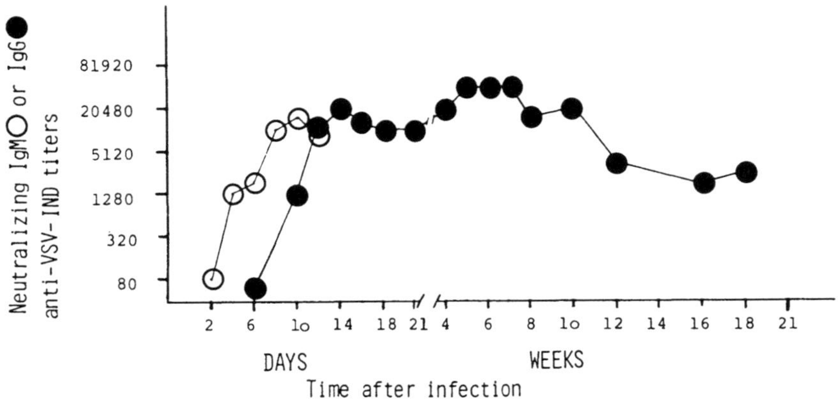


**Fig. 1.** Time course of a primary antibody response to VSV-IND. DBA/2 mice were infected with $2 \times 10^6$ pfu of VSV-IND. They were bled at the indicated times and neutralizing antibody titers were determined

were monitored. One may therefore argue that T-cell memory may be more quantitative than qualitative, in that relative precursor frequencies of relevant T cells are temporarily increased for a limited period and that rules established for anti-hapten antibody responses may not generally apply. This review is written from the infectious disease standpoint, using the premise that immunological memory is relevant only if it can function in a host, i.e., if it prevents disease caused by the same or by an immunologically cross-reactive, infectious agent. The collected evidence is presented from a biased point of view showing that, in contrast to B-cell memory, what we call T-cell memory may be rather limited in extent and duration.

## 2 Current Knowledge of the Kinetics of T-Cell Responses and Memory

T-cell responses against viruses or facultative intracellular bacteria are apparently rather short-lived (Blanden 1974; Doherty and Zinkernagel 1974). Antiviral cytolytic T lymphocyte (CTL) responses usually peak about 2–3 days after maximal virus titers and are not measurable beyond 3–5 days after viral titers fall below detectable levels (Fig. 2); the same is true for T-cell responses against facultative intracellular bacteria such as *Listeria monocytogenes* (Mackaness 1969; Jungi 1980).

If the kinetics of secondary antiviral T-cell responses are compared with the kinetics of primary responses, hardly any of the classic parameters of immunological memory are noticeable, i.e., there is little acceleration of the response—1/2 –

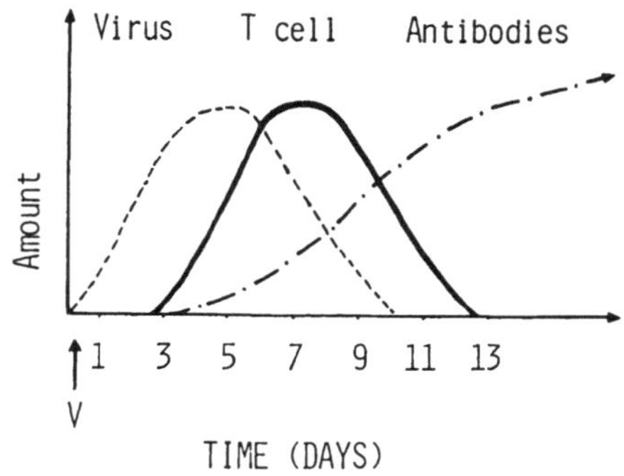


**Fig. 2.** Schematic representation of the kinetics of virus titers (*dashed line*) and cytotoxic T-cell (*solid line*) and antibody (*dotted-dashed line*) responses after i.v. injection of virus into a mouse

1 day—and no augmentation of the response (increased affinity cannot be assessed for T cells). This may be suggested by various published experiments on T-cell responses against arboviruses (WOLCOTT et al. 1982; MULLBACHER et al. 1981), influenza viruses (DOHERTY et al. 1977; TOWNSEND and MCMICHAEL 1985; MCMICHAEL et al. 1983), and *L. monocytogenes* (JUNGI 1980; MACKANESS 1969).

There is older evidence in the literature (PIRQUET 1907), and there are more recent World Health Organisation guidelines for vaccinations against pox virus, suggesting that T-cell-dependent memory (and protection against pox virus) may be rather short-lived. There is no doubt that vaccination with vaccinia virus does protect against systemic hematogenic spread of virus (as do most vaccinations) through induction of neutralizing antibodies; however, PIRQUET (1907) illustrated that virus-induced skin lesions develop comparably in both vaccinated and non-vaccinated individuals about 3–4 weeks after vaccination.

Admittedly, some findings from in vitro immunological studies do not readily fit the above bias, which is derived from experience in vivo e.g., unprimed lymphocytes cannot (BLANDEN et al. 1977) be triggered to make a measurable antiviral response in vitro, whereas primed ones can (PLATA et al. 1975). Whether this is due to (only temporary?) an increase of relative precursor frequencies alone or to the fact that culture conditions are still somewhat limited remains to be evaluated.

## 3 Antiviral Cytotoxic T-Cell Memory In Vivo

If mice are primed with vaccinia virus, vesicular stomatitis virus (VSV), or lymphocytic choriomeningitis virus (LCMV) and then challenged with the same virus, usually no appreciable CTL response can be measured during days 1–7 after challenge. If huge doses of virus are used for the challenge infection, a CTL response may be seen which exhibits kinetics not drastically different from the kinetics seen during a primary response. An example of this with VSV is shown in Fig. 3.

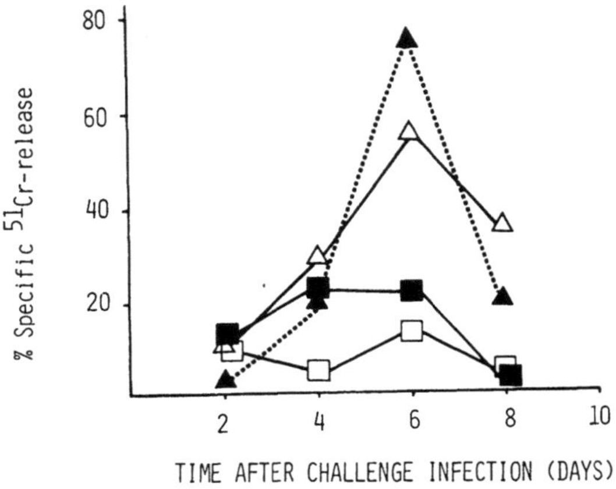


**Fig. 3.** C57BL/6 mice were injected with VSV-IND ($5 \times 10^6$ pfu) i.v. and challenged with $5 \times 10^9$ pfu VSV-IND 8 weeks later. Cytotoxic T-cell responses of these mice (*white symbols*) and of controls (*black symbols*) at the indicated times after the challenge infection on VSV-infected MC57G (H-$2^b$) target cells (*triangles*) or on NK-sensitive YAC cells (*squares*). The effector lymphocytes were also tested on uninfected MC57G cells but there was no significant release of $^{51}Cr$

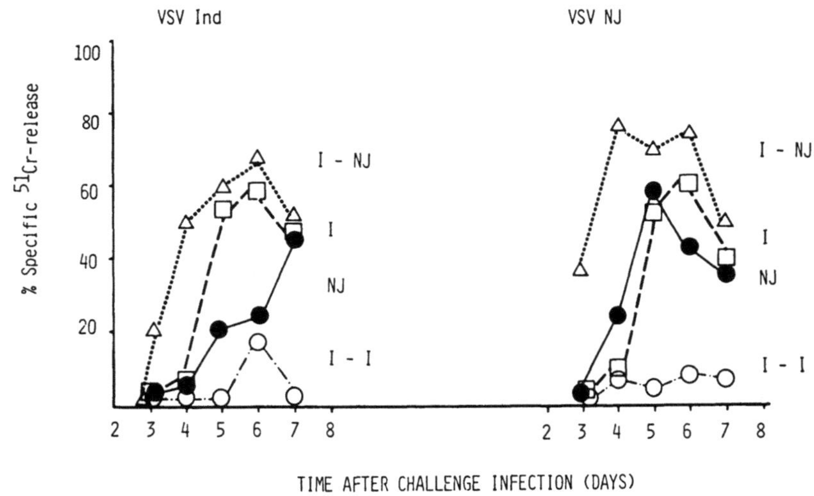


**Fig. 4.** C57BL/6 mice had been infected with about $5 \times 10^6$ pfu VSV-IND and were challenged 8 weeks later with $5 \times 10^6$ pfu of the same or the heterologous VSV. Cytotoxic T-cell responses were tested on VSV-IND (*left*, normal) or VSV-NJ (*right*) infected MC57G cells; no significant release of $^{51}Cr$ was found from uninfected target cells. *I-NJ*, mice primed with VSV-IND challenged with VSV-NJ (*triangles*); *I*, normal mice challenged with VSV-IND (*squares*); *NJ*, normal mice challenged with VSV-NJ (*circles*); *I-I*, mice primed with VSV-IND and challenged with VSV-IND (○)

Doses of virus which are more physiological may reveal comparable results if two separate viruses that are serologically distinct but share cross-reactive T-cell determinants are used for the priming and second challenge infection. DOHERTY and coworkers (EFFROS et al. 1978) have used two distinct influenza A strains to show an enhanced CTL response to the second challenge. We have chosen a similar approach using VSV-Indiana and -New Jersey (Fig. 4). Although a slight

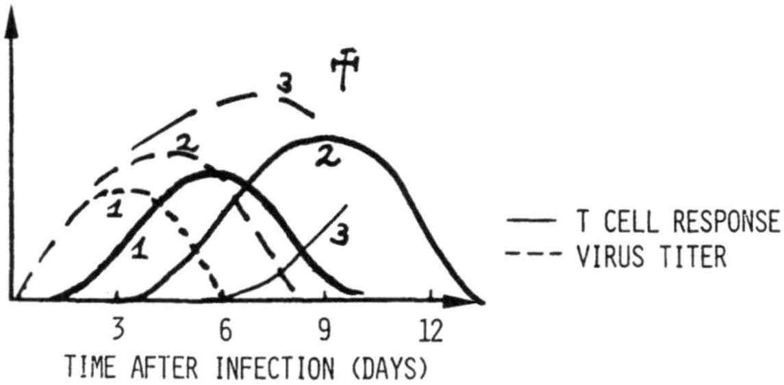


**Fig. 5.** Comparisons of the effects of three levels of preexistent or basic levels of T-cell immune responsiveness (*solid lines*) on the kinetics of virus titers *dashed lines*. The quicker and greater a T-cell immune response is, the less the virus can spread. Relatively small differences in the kinetics of the T-cell responses may have profound influences on virial kinetics; the cross in kinetics 3 indicates death of the host

acceleration might be seen during the early phase of induction of the secondary CTL response, the overall kinetics of the decline of the response are similar to those found in primary responses. It must be noted that this finding is best demonstrated if the virus dose used for the challenge infection is 20–100 times larger than that used to induce the primary response.

It should also be clearly stated here that, in operational terms, these experiments demonstrate functional T-cell memory; the fact that a host is capable of easily combatting an infectious dose that is 100 times greater than the dose usually needed to yield a comparable T-cell response is proof enough. The character of this memory may be readily explained by increased precursor frequencies. For example, a modest two- to eightfold increase of precursor effector cells would accelerate the efficient elimination of virus by 1–3 days compared with the elimination kinetics in an unprimed animal. This small difference in kinetics is usually sufficient to determine whether clinical disease is very limited and thus unapparent, or extensive and manifest (Fig. 5).

## 4 Studies on the Kinetics of Antiviral T-Helper Cells

### 4.1 The Experimental Rationale

Evidence has accumulated in recent years showing that T cells in general may be specific for processed antigens, i.e., antigen fragments rather than intact protein structures (Buus et al. 1987; Guillet et al. 1987; Babbitt et al. 1985; Germain 1986; Rock and Benacerraf 1983; Hackett et al. 1983; Kees and Krammer 1984; Townsend et al. 1986; Yewdell et al. 1985). Since serologically distinct but related viruses such as influenza viruses and VSVs apparently share many common determinants that may be recognized by T cells (Hackett et al. 1983;

KEES and KRAMMER 1984; TOWNSEND et al. 1986; MULLBACHER et al. 1981; WOLCOTT et al. 1982; YEWDELL et al. 1985; DOHERTY et al. 1977; ROSENTHAL and ZINKERNAGEL 1980; YEWDELL et al. 1986; ZINKERNAGEL and ROSENTHAL 1981), these findings raise the important question as to why immunological cross-protection is not much more efficiently mediated by cross-reactive cytotoxic or helper T cells in vivo (ANONYMOUS 1986; TOWNSEND and MCMICHAEL 1985; FAZEKAS DE ST. GROTH 1981; ANDREW et al. 1987; MULLBACHER et al. 1981; WOLCOTT et al. 1982; ZINKERNAGEL et al. 1985).

This question was analyzed by studying the T-help-dependent neutralizing anti-VSV antibody response to find whether there is cross-reactive T help in vivo after infection of mice with the two major serotypes of VSV. VSV is a bullet-shaped rhabdovirus carrying 8- to 10-nm-long glycoprotein spikes on its surface (WAGNER 1975). On the basis of neutralizing determinants located on these surface glycoproteins, two distinct serotypes have been identified, i.e., VSV-Indiana (IND) and VSV-New Jersey (NJ; DIETZSCHOLD et al. 1974). In addition, the glycoproteins of these two serotypes share some common epitopes (GALLIONE and ROSE 1983) which have been confirmed by analysis with monoclonal antibodies (LEFRANCOIS and LYLES 1982a, b; BRICKER et al. 1987; GALLIONE and ROSE 1983). Shared common determinants on the nucleoprotein and to a lesser extent on the glycoprotein may be recognized by cross-reactive VSV-specific CTLs (ROSENTHAL and ZINKERNAGEL 1980; YEWDELL et al. 1986) and possibly also by helper T cells (RUSSELL and LIEW 1980; LAMB et al. 1982; THOMAS et al. 1972).

## 4.2 Priming of Mice with VSV-IND Fails to Enhance a Neutralizing Response to VSV-NJ But Enhances the Anti-DNP Response to VSV-NJ-DNP

It is well documented that cooperation between T and B cells is necessary for induction of antibodies to T-dependent antigens (SWAIN 1981; KATZ and BENACERRAF 1972); this need is absolute for the induction of neutralizing IgG responses to VSV (CHARAN and ZINKERNAGEL 1986). Priming of mice with one serotype of VSV 20 weeks prior to challenging prepared the animals to respond to a second infection with heterologous VSV with an enhanced and accelerated secondary type of antibody response in vivo. This response was measured by an antibody binding assay (ELISA) but was not evident when monitored by a virus neutralization assay (Fig. 6; GUPTA et al. 1986).

Mice were primed with live or UV-inactivated VSV-IND serotype (Fig. 7) with or without (not shown) complete Freund's adjuvant (GUPTA et al. 1986). After challenge with VSV-NJ, these mice developed a secondary-type IgG response, measured by antibody binding in an ELISA, against both VSV-IND and VSV-NJ. The same result was found for the reciprocal experiments where mice were primed with VSV-NJ. Similarly, when mice were primed with live VSV, UV-inactivated VSV, or purified VSV glycoprotein of IND or NJ serotype and

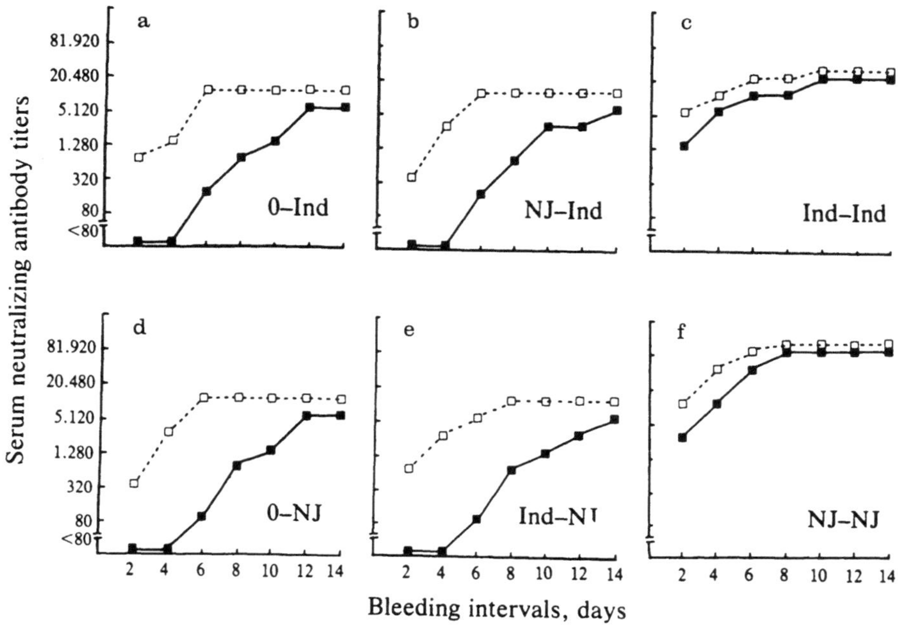


**Fig. 6a–f.** Anti-VSV-IND (**a–c**) and anti-VSV-NJ (**d–f**) serum neutralizing antibody responses in mice. *Solid squares*, IgG titers; *open squares*, total IgM + IgG antibody titers. **a, d** anti-VSV serum neutralizing antibody kinetics in unprimed mice. Anti-VSV kinetics in mice primed 22 weeks earlier with VSV-NJ (**b**) or VSV-IND (**e**) and challenged with the heterologous serotype. Anti-VSV kinetics in mice primed 22 weeks earlier with VSV-IND (**c**) or VSV-NJ (**f**) and challenged with the homologous serotype. Antibody titers before challenge at 22 weeks were 1:1280 (from GUPTA et al. 1986)

challenged later with dinitrophenyl (DNP)-conjugated, UV-inactivated VSV or with DNP-conjugated glycoprotein of either serotype, they exhibited a secondary-type anti-DNP antibody response which was demonstrated by the binding of IgG to dinitrophenylated bovine serum albumin and measured by ELISA (Fig. 7; GUPTA et al. 1986). In contrast, when neutralizing antibody responses were monitored, VSV-IND-primed mice challenged with VSV-NJ developed a strictly primary-type anti-VSV-NJ response, and vice versa. Thus, preexisting helper T cells specific for shared carrier determinants do not improve virign B-cell responses specific for "new" unique determinants that are the targets for the biologically relevant neutralizing antibodies. These findings and those showing an apparent absence of cross-protection in vivo can be explained by postulating that only T cells specific for nonshared distinct determinants on antigen fragments or protein structures are protective, or that a special requirement exists favoring collaborations between neighboring B- and T-cell epitopes (MANCA et al. 1985; BERZOFSKY 1983). In addition, B-cell frequency and response, and not T help, may be the limiting factor for cross-protection. Alternatively, functional T helper cells may be short-lived in vivo, or

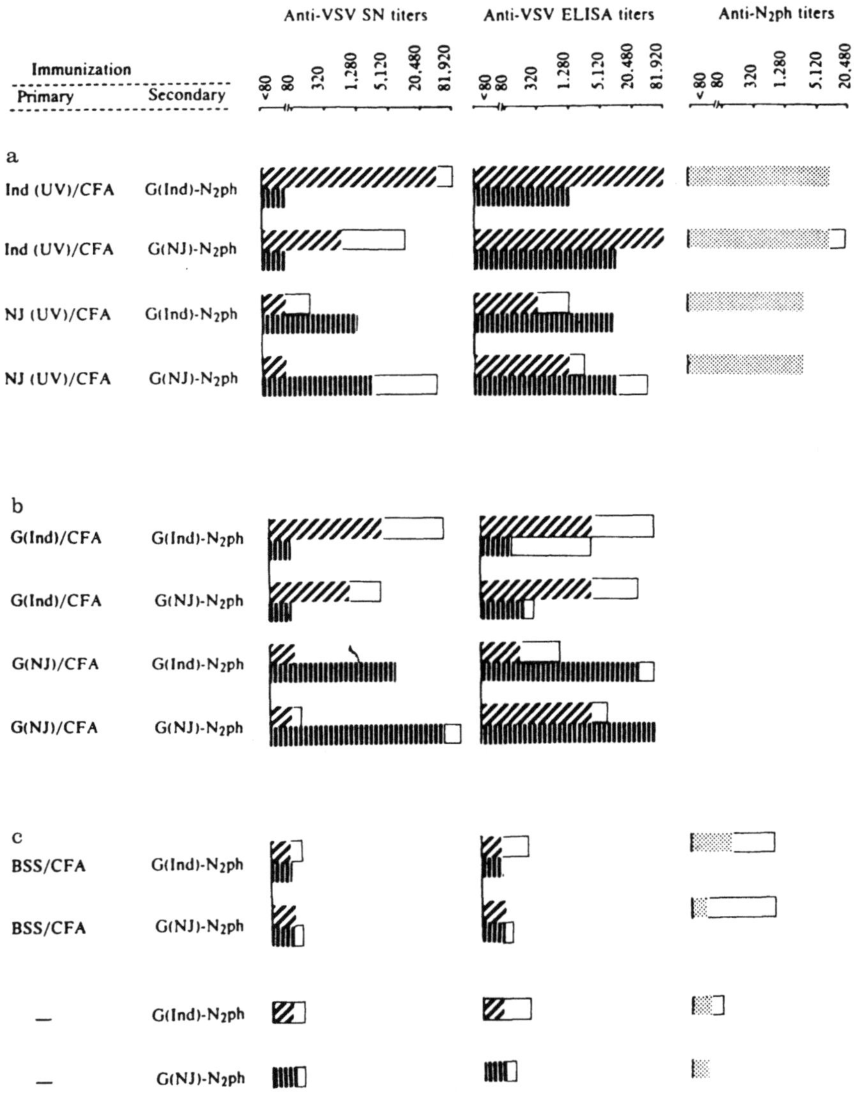


**Fig. 7 a–c.** Capacity of VSV-IND and VSV-NJ viral antigens to function as carrier molecules. Mice were primed with $10^8$ pfu of UV-inactivated VSV-IND or VSV-NJ in CFA and injected i.v. 3 weeks later with 20 μg IND-DNP (*IND-$N_2pH$*) or NJ-DNP (*NJ-$N_2pH$*) in Hanks balanced salts solutions (*BSS*). Sera were obtained on days 4 and 8 after secondary immunization. Anti-VSV-IND IgG antibody titers (*diagonally hatched bars*) and anti-VSV-NJ IgG antibody titers (*hatched bars*) were detected by serum neutralization (*SN*) test and ELISA, and anti-DNP ($N_2$ph) titers (*stippled bars*) were measured by ELISA. Titers on day 4 are shown by *hatched* or *stippled bars*, and increased titers on day 8, by *extended open bars* (from Gupta et al. 1986)

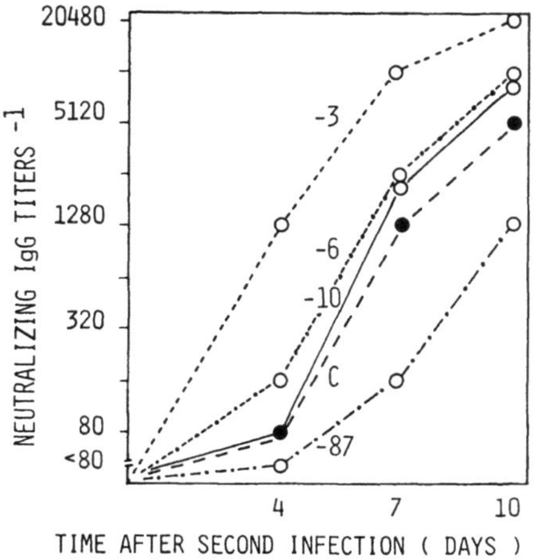


**Fig. 8.** Effect of priming with heterologous serotype on CS-A resistant anti-VSV-NJ neutralizing IgG responses. Groups of three to four mice primed 3, 6, 10, or 87 days earlier with VSV-IND (2 × $10^6$ pfu i.v.) were given a second infection with VSV-NJ (2 × $10^6$ pfu i.v.) and treated daily with CS-A (60 mg/kg) (*open circles*); additional unprimed control mice were not treated with CS-A (*solid circles*). Neutralizing IgG titers against the second infection were assayed on days 4, 7, and 10. Unprimed mice treated with CS-A and challenged with VSV-NJ (not shown) showed no measurable IgG response (from S. CHARAN et al., unpublished observations)

perhaps primed cross-reactive T help is difficult to recruit (JUNGI 1980; SPRENT and MILLER 1976).

## 4.3 Kinetics of T Help Cross-Reacting Between VSV-IND and VSV-NJ

To evaluate the kinetics of functional effector and memory T help in vivo, the effect of priming with one serotype of VSV-IND on the antibody response to a serologically distinct heterologous second serotype was studied (H.P. ROOST et al., unpublished observations). Mice primed with VSV-IND for 3 or 6 days, but not those primed for 17 or more days, showed an earlier and enhanced IgG response to neutralizing determinants of VSV-NJ than unprimed controls (Table 1). Thus, cross-reactive T help may be operative in vivo but apparently can only be

**Table 1.** Kinetics of the enhanced neutralizing IgG response to VSV-NJ after priming of mice with VSV-IND

| Time between priming infections with VSV-IND and challenge infection (days) | Neutralizing IgG anti-VSV-NJ titers on day 6 after challenge infection |
|---|---|
| 3 | 1:160 |
| 6 | 1:320 |
| 17 | 1:80 |
| 85 | < 1:80 |
| Unprimed control | < 1:80 |

DBA/2 mice were primed with 2 × $10^6$ pfu of VSV-IND and challenged with 2 × $10^6$ pfu of VSV-NJ. Adapted from H.P. ROOST et al. (unpublished observations)

demonstrated for a limited time with the readout used (Charan et al. 1988).

Kinetics of memory T help in vivo were also analyzed with the help of cyclosporin A (CS-A). Doses 30–60 mg/kg CS-A per day were necessary for suppression of primary anti-VSV IgG antibody responses when CS-A treatment was started on day 0. When daily CS-A treatment (60 mg/kg per day) was started on various later days, induction of the neutralizing IgG anti-VSV response was suppressed only if CS-A treatment was started before day 3–4. These results demonstrate that the kinetics of induction of specific T-helper cells follow the rapid time course kinetics of CTLs. Mice primed with VSV-IND, when given a second infection with heterologous VSV-NJ along with CS-A (60 mg/kg per day) up to 6 months later, were able to respond with a neutralizing IgG response that was however strictly of the primary type, whereas unprimed mice otherwise treated identically were unable to do so. Thus, mice primed with one serotype could provide T help during a response against the heterologous serotype even if treated with CS-A, and this CS-A-resistant T help was long-lived but not able to enhance a primary B-cell response. The kinetics of the capacity of CS-A-resistant T helper cells to enhance the IgG antibody response against a second infection with the heterologous VSV, as compared to a normal primary response, were studied using this protocol. An enhancing CS-A-resistant cross-reactive T helper effect was found 3–10 days after priming. This enhancing cross-reactive T help was as short-lived as primary virus-specific cytotoxic T-cell responses: it peaked around 3–8 days and was demonstrable only up to 2 weeks after priming (H.P. Roost et al., unpublished observations). Thus, there exists an experimentally demonstrable T helper cell memory that can be induced in vitro or shown to function under CS-A treatment in vivo and which seems to persist in mice for many months. This T-helper cell memory is apparently not functionally able to improve B-cell responses in vivo over those seen during a conventional primary response later than about 2–3 weeks after induction.

As discussed before, this may be due to the small number of precursor B cells which limit the primary response, rather than due to inefficiently primed cross-reactive T-help. If protective antiviral transplantation-antigen-restricted T cells recognize fragments of antigens shared between serologically distinct viruses, both short half life of T help and low precursor frequencies of B cells could explain why T-cell-mediated cross-protection against serologically distinct but closely related viruses could not efficiently prevent viral replication 2–4 weeks after infection. If these findings can be further supported and generalized, they must be considered when vaccine strategies are planned.

## 5 Conclusion

Both the differing specificities of antiviral antibody responses versus T-cell responses and the differences in B-cell memory and persistence of an antibody response versus the shorter-lived kinetics of T-cell memory may be a reflection of the balanced relationship between infectious agents and vertebrate hosts (ZINKERNAGEL et al. 1985). The question as to why long-lasting B-cell memory apparently exists in contrast to the possibly limited T-cell memory remains unanswered. Is it because antibodies and B cells form a circular system as speculated in the network hypotheses or, more likely, is it because antibodies but not T cells are vertically transmitted from mother to offspring (ZINKERNAGEL et al. 1985)? T cells, the phylogenetically older part of the immune system which cannot be transmitted from mother to offspring, may have to be in maximal and optimal condition at all times. What benefit would immunological memory be if the host were killed during a primary infection? Thus, T-cell responses against intracellular parasites must be as efficient and as rapid as possible.

The most important practical implications of the arguments presented are obvious. Firstly, antibodies or T cells are efficient only against determinants that can be appropriately recognized for topographical reasons. Protection by antibodies can be provided only against determinants that are properly exposed under physiological conditions. Therefore, probably only a few possible determinants synthesized by conventional protein synthesis or by using DNA-technology will prove helpful when preparing vaccines; additionally, it is not easily conceivable that "new" relevant and protective determinants will be found by such methods. Secondly, protection by vaccination which induces T-cell responses may prove difficult because its efficiency depends upon many different determinants being presented by the vaccine so that major histocompatibility complex (MHC)-dependent antigen presentation can be optimal for the species and because the protection may possibly be rather short-lived. Biologically important, long-lasting protection may then be more readily provided by proper antibodies and B-cell memory which is of the correct class and location.

## References


Andrew ME, Coupar BEH, Boyle DB, Ada GL (1987) The roles of influenza virus haemagglutinin and nucleoprotein in protection: analysis using vaccinia virus recombinants. Scand J Immunol 25: 21–28

Anonymous (1986) Reinfections with influenza. Lancet ii: 372–374

Babbitt BP, Allen PM, Matsueda G, Haber E, Unanue ER (1985) Binding of immunogenic peptides to Ia histocompatibility molecules. Nature 317: 359–360

Berzofsky JA (1983) T-B reciprocity: an Ia-restricted epitopes-specific circuit regulating T cell-B cell interaction and antibody specificity. Surv Immunol Res 2: 223–230

Blanden RV (1974) T cell response to viral and bacterial infection. Transplant Rev 19: 56–84

Blanden RV, Kees U, Dunlop MBC (1977) In vitro primary induction of cytotoxic T cells against virus-infected syngeneic cells. J Immunol Methods 16: 73–89

Bricker BJ, Snyder RM, Fox JW, Volk WA, Wagner RR (1987) Monoclonal antibodies to the glycoprotein of vesicular stomatitis virus (New Jersey Serotype): a method for preliminary mapping of epitopes. Virology 161: 533–540

Buus S, Sette A, Colon SM, Miles C, Grey HM (1987) The relation between major histocompatibility complex (MHC) restriction and the capacity of Ia to bind immunogenic peptides. Science 235: 1353–1358

Charan S, Zinkernagel RM (1986) Antibody mediated suppression of secondary IgM response in nude mice against vesicular stomatitis virus. J Immunol 136: 3057–3061
Charan S, Roost HP, Hengartner H, Zinkernagel RM (1989) Analysis of the kinetics of antiviral T help in vivo (manuscript in preparation)
Dietzschold B, Schneider LG, Cox JH (1974) Serological characterization of the three major proteins of vesicular stomatitis virus. J Virol 14: 1–7
Doherty PC, Zinkernagel RM (1974) T cell-mediated immunopathology in viral infection. Transplant Rev 19: 89–120
Doherty PC, Effros RB, Bennink J (1977) Heterogeneity of the cytotoxic response of thymus-derived lymphocytes after immunization with influenza viruses. Proc Natl Acad Sci USA 74: 1209–1213
Effors RB, Bennink J, Doherty PC (1978) Characteristics of secondary cytotoxic T cell responses in mice infected with influenza A virus. Cell Immunol 36: 345–353
Fazekas de St. Groth S (1981) The joint evolution of antigens and antibodies in the immune system. In: Steinberg CM, Lefkovits I (eds) The immune system, Vol. I. Karger, Basel, pp 155–168
Gallione CJ, Rose JK (1983) Nucleotide sequence of a cDNA clone encoding the entire glycoprotein from the New Jersey serotype of vesicular stomatitis virus. J Virol 46: 162–169
Germain RN (1986) The ins and outs of antigen processing and presentation. Nature 322: 687–689
Guillet JG, Lai M-Z, Briner TJ, Buus S, Sette A, Grey HM, Smith JA, Gefter ML (1987) Immunological self, nonself discrimination. Science 235: 865–870
Gupta SC, Hengartner H, Zinkernagel RM (1986) Primary antibody responses to a well-defined and unique hapten are not enhanced by preimmunization with carrier: analysis in a viral model. Proc Natl Acad Sci USA 83: 2604–2608
Hackett CJ, Dietzschold B, Gerhard W, Ghrist B, Knorr R, Gillessen D, Melchers F (1983) Influenza virus site recognized by a murine helper T cell specific for H1 strains: localisation to a nine amino acid sequence in the hemagglutinin molecule. J Exp Med 158: 294–302
Jungi TW (1980) Immunological memory to *Listeria monocytogenes* in rodents: evidence for protective T lymphocytes outside the recirculating lymphocyte pool. J Reticuloendothel Soc 28: 405–417
Katz DH (1977) Lymphocyte differentiation, recognition and regulation. Academic, New York
Katz DH, Benacerraf B (1972) The regulatory influence of activated T cells on B cell responses to antigens. Adv Immunol 15: 1–94
Kees U, Krammer PH (1984) Most influenza A virus specific memory cytotoxic T lymphocytes react with antigenic epitopes associated with internal virus determinants. J Exp Med 159: 365–377
Lamb JR, Eckles DD, Lake P, Woody JN, Green N (1982) Human T-cell clones recognize chemically synthesized peptides of influenza hemagglutinin. Nature 300: 66–69
Lefrançois L, Lyles DS (1982a) The interaction of antibody with the major surface glycoprotein of vesicular stomatitis virus. II. Monoclonal antibodies to non-neutralizing and cross-reactive epitopes of Indiana and New Jersey serotypes. Virology 121: 168–174
Lefrançois L, Lyles DS (1982b) The interaction of antibody with the major surface glycoprotein of vesicular stomatitis virus. I. Analysis of neutralizing epitopes with monoclonal antibodies. Virology 121: 157–167
Mackaness GB (1969) The influence of immunologically committed lymphoid cells on macrophage activity in vivo. J Exp Med 129: 973–992
Manca F, Kunkl A, Fenoglio D, Fowler A, Sercarz E, Celada F (1985) Constraints in T-B cooperation related to epitope topology on *E. coli* $\beta$-galactosidase. – I. The fine specificity of T cells dictates the fine specificity of antibodies directed to conformation-dependent determinants. Eur J Immunol 15: 345–350
McMichael AJ, Gotch FM, Dongworth DW, Clark A, Potter C (1983) Declining T cell immunity to influenza 1977–1982. Lancet ii: 762–764
Mullbacher A, Marshall ID, Blanden RV (1981) Cross-reactive cytotoxic T cell to alphavirus infection. Scand J Immunol 10: 291–297
Pirquet C (1907) Von klinischen Studien über Vakzination und vakzinale Allergie. Denticke, F Leipzig
Plata F, Cerottini JC, Brunner KT (1975) Primary and secondary in vitro generation of cytolytic T lymphocytes in the murine sarcoma virus system. Eur J Immunol 5: 227–233
Rock KL, Benacerraf B (1983) Inhibition of antigen-specific T lymphocyte activation by structurally related Ir gene-controlled polymers. J Exp Med 157: 1618–1634
Rosenthal KL, Zinkernagel RM (1980) Cross-reactive cytotoxic T cells to serologically distinct vesicular stomatitis viruses. J Immunol 124: 2301–2308

Russell SM, Liew FY (1980) Cell cooperation in antibody responses to influenza virus. I. Priming of helper T cells by internal components of the virion. Eurr J Immunol. 10: 791–796
Sprent J, Miller JFAP (1976) Effect of recent antigen priming on adoptive immune responses. III. Antigen-induced selective recruitment of subsets of recirculating lymphocytes reactive to H-2 determinants. J Exp Med 143: 585–598
Swain SL (1981) Significance of Lyt phenotypes: Lyt-2 antibodies block activities of T cells that recognize class I major histocompatibility complex antigens regardless of their function. Proc Natl Acad Sci USA 78: 7101–7105
Thomas DB, Hackett CJ, Askonas BA (1972) Evidence for two T-helper populations with distinct specificity in the humoral response to influenza A viruses. Immunology 47: 429–436
Townsend ARM, McMichael AJ (1985) Specificity of cytotoxic T lymphocytes stimulated with influenza virus. Studies in mice and humans. Prog Allergy 36: 10–43
Townsend ARM, Rothbard J, Gotch FM, Bahadur G, Wraith D, McMichael AJ (1986) The epitopes of influenza nucleoprotein recognized by cytotoxic T lymphocytes can be defined with short synthetic peptides. Cell 44: 959–968
Wagner RR (1975) Reproduction of rhabdoviruses: composite model of infection. Virology 4: 41
Wolcott JA, Wust CJ, Brown A (1982) Immunization with one alphavirus cross-primes cellular and humoral immune responses to a second alphavirus. J Immunol 129: 1267–1271
Yewdell JW, Bennink JR, Smith GL, Moss B (1985) Influenza A virus nucleoprotein is a major target antigen for cross-reactive anti-influenza A virus nucleoprotein is a major target antigen for cross-reactive anti-influenza A virus cytotoxic T lymphocytes. Proc Natl Acad Sci USA 82: 1785–1789
Yewdell JW, Bennink JR, Mackett M, Lefrançois L, Lyles DS, Moss B (1986) Recognition of cloned vesicular stomatitis virus internal and external gene products by cytotoxic T lymphocytes. J Exp Med 163: 1529–1538
Zinkernagel RM (1979) Heterogeneization and MHC restricted T cells. In: Kobayashi H (ed) Immunological zenogenization of tumor cells. University Park Press, Baltimore, pp 181–184
Zinkernagel RM, Rosenthal KL (1981) Experiments and speculation on antiviral specificity of T and B cells. Immunol Rev 58: 131–155
Zinkernagel RM, Hengartner H, Stitz L (1985) On the role of viruses in the evolution of immune responses. Br Med Bull 41: 92–97

# Subsets of Rat CD4$^+$ T Cells Defined by Their Differential Expression of Variants of the CD45 Antigen: Developmental Relationships and In Vitro and In Vivo Functions

F. POWRIE and D. MASON



## 1 Introduction

Thymus-derived lymphocytes have been shown to mediate a wide range of immunological functions both as direct effectors in cell-mediated immunity and as helper or inducer cells for B cells, macrophages, bone marrow cells and other T cells. In addition, the lymphokines that they produce have been shown to act not only on leucocytes but also on non-bone marrow derived cells. This wide range of T-cell functions has only recently been fully appreciated, but early work using alloantisera in mice established that T cells with different functional specializations could be distinguished phenotypically on the basis of whether or not they expressed what came to be called the CD8 antigen (CANTOR and BOYSE 1975).

With the development of monoclonal antibodies and their rapid application to the study of T-cell heterogeneity (WILLIAMS et al. 1977; MASON et al. 1980;

Medical Research Council Cellular Immunology Unit, Sir William Dunn School of Pathology, University of Oxford, South Parks Road, Oxford, OX1 3RE, United Kingdom

Current Topics in Microbiology and Immunology, Vol. 159

REINHERZ and SCHLOSSMAN 1980), it became apparent that peripheral T cells could be divided into two major groups, those that expressed the CD4 antigen and those that expressed CD8. However, a number of monoclonal antibodies that recognize different forms of the leucocyte-common antigen, CD45, are now available. These demonstrate further phenotypic heterogeneity within these two major subsets of T cells (SPICKETT et al. 1983; MORIMOTO et al. 1985; TERRY et al. 1988), and these findings raise the question as to whether or not such phenotypic heterogeneity is related to further functional specialization. This review describes experiments designed to study this question.

## 2 Heterogeneity of the CD45 Antigen

All leucocytes in man (DALCHAU et al. 1980), mouse (TROWBRIDGE 1978) and rat (STANDRING et al. 1978) express a major membrane glycoprotein of approximately 200 kD. Historically this molecule has been given different names in the three species: CD45 in man (COBBOLD et al. 1987), T200 in the mouse (TROWBRIDGE et al. 1977) and the leucocyte-common antigen (LCA) in the rat (FABRE and WILLIAMS 1977). In keeping with our general practice of using the cluster of differentiation (CD) terminology wherever amino acid or DNA sequencing data establish interspecies homologies, we shall refer to the rat molecule as CD45. Molecular weight determinations have revealed that the CD45 antigen exists in several different forms in all three species. In the rat, for example, the CD45 antigen isolated from purified subpopulations of lymphocytes produces discrete bands on polyacrylamide gel electrophoresis (PAGE) that correspond to molecular weights of 180, 190, 200, 220 and 240 kDa. As Table 1 shows, the actual bands obtained depend on the cell type from which the CD45 antigen is obtained. The 240-kD form is particularly heterogeneous in apparent molecular weight but this is less so for the lower molecular weight components. Nevertheless there is serological evidence that there is more heterogeneity than the gel electrophoresis suggests, since a monoclonal antibody MRC OX-22 that reacts with components

**Table 1.** Molecular weight heterogeneity of CD45 found on rat lymphocyte subpopulations

| Lymphocyte subset | Apparent $M_r \times 10^{-3}$ |
|---|---|
| B cells | 240 |
| CD4 T cells | 180, 190, 200, 220 |
| CD8 T cells | 180, 190, 200, 220 |
| Thymocytes | 180, 190 |

The molecular weight of the CD45 antigen was determined by sodium dodecyl sulphate (SDS) PAGE of lymphoid cell surface glycoproteins purified on an MRC OX-1 column. (WOOLLETT et al. 1985)

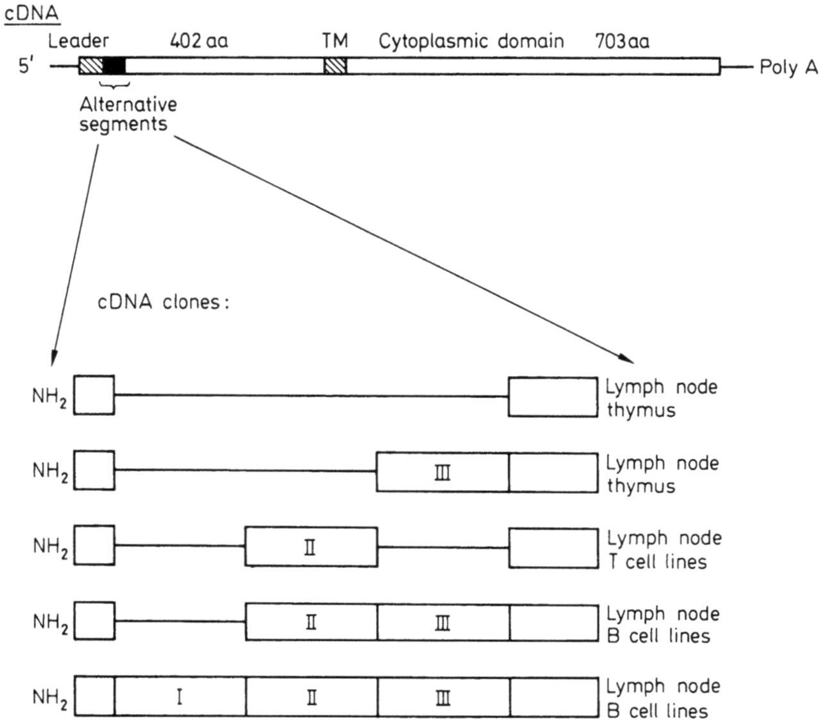


**Fig. 1.** Alternative splicing of the CD45 molecule (LCA). The CD45 molecule spans the cell membrane to yield a cytoplasmic domain of 703 amino acids (*aa*) and an extracellular part with 402 or more amino acids (THOMAS et al. 1985). Different cDNA clones of CD45 have different sequences at the 5′ end. The five clones which have been sequenced are shown in exploded view. All five forms have not been found in any one species. The form expressing exon III alone has been found only in the mouse (SAGA et al. 1987) and rat (BARCLAY et al. 1987) whereas that expressing exons II and III (SAGA et al. 1987; STREULI et al. 1987a) has been found in both mouse and human but not in the rat. The other three forms shown are common to all three species. The tissue from which the library was obtained is noted next to the form of the cDNA clone sequenced

of all the forms except the 180-kD one, seems to precipitate only some of the material in these higher molecular weight bands (WOOLLETT et al. 1985).

Studies of complementary (c)DNA clones and genomic DNA in rat (BARCLAY et al. 1987), human (RALPH et al. 1987) and mouse (THOMAS et al. 1987; SAGA et al. 1987) have shown that there is amino acid sequence variation near the $NH_2$-terminus of the CD45 molecule and that this variation, which accounts for the multiple bands seen on gel electrophoresis, arises because three different exons code for the sequence of this part of the molecule (Fig. 1). Differential splicing of RNA can, in principle, produce eight different forms of the molecule, and although it is not known how many actually are produced the number is at least five since this number of cDNA clones have been isolated (BARCLAY et al. 1987; RALPH et al. 1987; THOMAS et al. 1987; SAGA et al. 1987; STREULI et al. 1987a). This finding provides a possible explanation for the serological data already

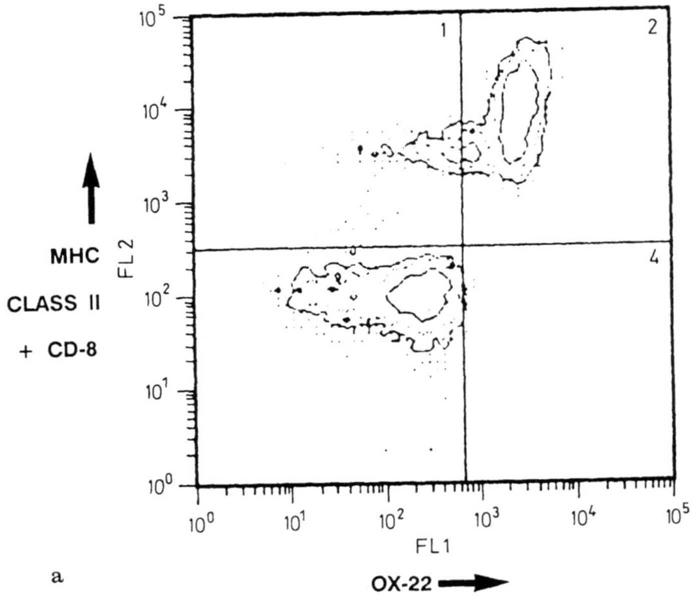


a

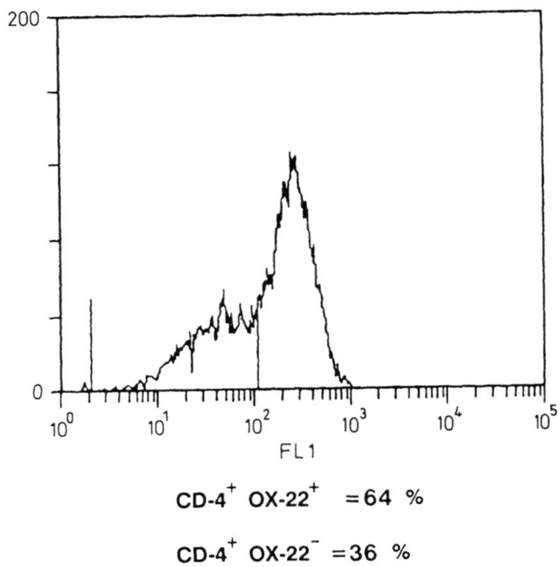


b

**Fig. 2 a, b.** Phenotypes of CD4$^+$ T cells shown by two-colour indirect immunofluorescent staining of rat TDL (MASON et al. 1987). **A** The X axis represents binding of OX-22 monoclonal antibody (mAb) expressed as the logarithm of green fluorescence and the Y axis represents binding of anti-class II, anti-immunoglobulin κ-chain and anti-CD8 mAbs expressed as the logarithm of red fluorescence. **B** OX-22 labelling pattern of the CD4$^+$ TDL. These cells were selected by gating out CD8$^+$, class II$^+$ and surface Ig$^+$ cells mentioned. In fact monoclonal antibodies to the CD45 antigen from rat and man that react with only some of the molecular weight forms of this antigen do so because they recognize products of the exons responsible for sequence near the $NH_2$-terminus. It is known, for example, that expression of exon I is not required to generate the determinant recognized by OX-22 antibody (Barclay et al. 1987). Similarly, monoclonal antibody 2H4 binds only to those components of human CD45 that use exon I (Streuli et al. 1987b). Another antibody, UCHLI, reacts only with the 180-kDa form of human CD45 and in this form none of the three exons are expressed (Streuli et al. 1988). This result explains the finding that 2H4 antibody does not react with the 180-kDa form of human CD45 antigen (Terry et al. 1988).

## 3 Differential Expression of Various Forms of the CD45 Antigen on $CD4^+$ T Cells

The use of monoclonal antibodies that recognize only some forms of rat or human CD45 antigen has proved invaluable in studying functional heterogeneity among $CD4^+$ T cells. The OX-22 antibody reacts with about 60%–70% of rat $CD4^+$ T cells (Fig. 2), and a rather smaller percentage of human $CD4^+$ cells in peripheral blood express the 2H4 antigenic determinant. As noted, the OX-22 antigen is found on some of the $190^-$, $200^-$, and 220-kDa components of rat CD45 (but not the 180-kDa one), and 2H4 antibody binds to the $200^-$ and $220^-$ kDa forms of the human molecule (Streuli et al. 1987b). Although these biochemical data suggested originally that the $OX\text{-}22^-$ $CD4^+$ T cells in rat and $2H4^-$ $CD4^+$ T cells in man are equivalent populations the more recent demonstration that antibodies OX-22 and 2H4 recognise different exon products of the CD45 gene, raises the possibility that this conclusion is not correct. In fact it is now known that the $2H4^-$ $CD4^+$ T cell subset can be further subdivided into two mutually exclusive populations that express different levels of exon II of human CD45, and the $OX\text{-}22^-$ $CD4^+$ T cells in the rat correspond to one of these (Mason and Powrie, submitted).

## 4 Tissue Distribution of the CD45 Molecule and OX-22 Determinant

As already noted, the CD45 molecule is found on all rat leucocytes (including thymocytes) and on no other cell types (Woollett et al. 1985). In contrast, the OX-22 determinant has a more restricted tissue distribution and the data are summarized in Table 2. It will be noted that, whereas all B cells appear to be

**Table 2.** Tissue distribution of those components of rat CD45 antigen that express the OX-22 epitope

| Cell type | Percentage cells labelled |
|---|---|
| B cells | 100 |
| Y3 rat myeloma | 0 |
| $CD4^+$ T cells | 50–75 |
| $CD8^+$ T cells (non-activated) | 100 |
| $CD4^+$ T-cell lines | 0 |
| $CD8^+$ cytotoxic T cells | 0 |
| Bone marrow cells | 50 |
| Thymocytes | ~2 |
| Polymorphonuclear | |
| Granulocytes | 0 |
| Natural killer cells | At least the majority |

The tissue distribution of cells binding OX-22 antibody was determined by analysis of FACS fluorescent histograms as previously described (SPICKETT et al. 1983)

$OX-22^+$, the rat myeloma Y3 does not express this determinant. It has also recently been demonstrated that normal rat plasma cells are $OX-22^-$ (B. VONDERHEIDE, personal communication).

## 5 Studies on the Functions of $OX-22^+$ $CD4^+$ and $OX-22^-$ $CD4^+$ T Cells

### 5.1 In Vivo

Experiments have been carried out to establish the OX-22 antigen phenotype of the $CD4^+$ T cell that provides help to antigen-primed B cells in secondary antibody responses and of the $CD4^+$ T cells that mediate in vivo alloreactivity, as judged by the popliteal lymph node assay (FORD et al. 1970) and the ability to induce fatal graft-versus-host disease.

To assess helper activity, thoracic duct lymphocytes (TDL) were obtained from donor rats primed 4–6 weeks earlier with dinitrophenyl-bovine $\gamma$-globulin (DNP-BGG). These TDL were separated by rosette depletion (MASON et al. 1987) and by the use of a fluorescence-activated cell sorter (FACS) into B cells and $OX-22^+$ $CD4^+$ and $OX-22^-$ $CD4^+$ T cells. Appropriate mixtures of primed B cells and subsets of $CD4^+$ T cells were injected, together with a challenge dose of DNP-BGG, into sublethally irradiated recipients, and anti-DNP antibody titres were measured by solid phase radioimmunoassay in sera obtained 7 days after cell transfer. The experiments showed that the $OX-22^-$ $CD4^+$ T-cell subset was far more potent than the $OX-22^+$ $CD4^+$ subset in providing help for B cells (SPICKETT et al. 1983). Since unprimed T cells (at the cell dose used) do not provide detectable help in this assay, it was concluded that most if not all memory helper T cells in this system were $OX-22^-$ $CD4^+$.

In contrast, cells of this phenotype showed no alloreactivity by either the popliteal lymph node or graft-versus-host assays, whereas the responses from the OX-22$^+$ CD4$^+$ T cells were not significantly different to those obtained from unfractionated CD4$^+$ cells (Spickett et al. 1983). These results on alloreactivity will be referred to again later in this review.

## 5.2 In Vitro

In vivo experiments, while physiologically more satisfactory than in vitro experiments, do not permit one to measure possible lymphokine production. For this reason a series of experiments were carried out in vitro to assess the functional capacities of both OX-22$^+$ and OX-22$^-$ subsets of CD4$^+$ T cells and to measure the levels of interleukin-2 that the two subsets produced on activation.

The studies on the helper activity of the two T-cell subsets confirmed the in vivo data in that culture wells that contained primed B cells and antigen were found to contain specific antibody only if OX-22$^-$ CD4$^+$ T cells from antigen-primed donors were also included in the culture. In this assay OX-22$^+$ CD4$^+$ cells were completely inert. However, this latter subset, unlike the OX-22$^-$ CD4$^+$ cells, responded vigorously in the mixed leucocyte culture and to the T-cell mitogen concanavalin A (Con A), and both forms of stimulus induced the OX-22$^+$ subset to produce interleukin-2 in readily detectable amounts. Little or no interleukin-2 was detected from wells containing OX-22$^-$ CD4$^+$ T cells even when the cells were demonstrably providing help for B cells (Arthur and Mason 1986). It was concluded from these experiments that the subset of CD4$^+$ T cells that made interleukin-2 was phenotypically distinguishable from the one that provided help for B cells in secondary antibody responses in vitro (Arthur and Mason 1986).

More recent work on the in vitro response of the OX-22$^-$ CD4$^+$ T-cell subset to alloantigens in mixed lymphocyte culture (MLC) has confirmed the earlier finding that this subset responds very poorly in these assays when, as in the original experiments, the culture medium contains 5% normal rat serum[1]. Unexpectedly, when the rat serum was replaced by fetal calf serum the OX-22$^-$ subset of CD4$^+$ cells proliferated as well as the OX-22$^+$ subset, both in response to Con A (Fig. 3a) and in the MLC (Fig. 3c). However, differences between the two populations were still apparent: measurements of interleukin-2 in the culture supernatants in these experiments demonstrated that, even in fetal calf serum, the OX-22$^-$ CD4$^+$ T cells produced very low levels of lymphokine compared with the OX-22$^+$ subset. (Fig. 3b, d). Rodent sera have been shown to contain

[1] It has been found that the response of the OX-22$^-$ CD4$^+$ cells in the MLC depends on the batch of rat serum used. Not all batches are strongly inhibitory of the response of this subset but no batch has been found that inhibits the OX-22$^+$ CD4$^+$ population

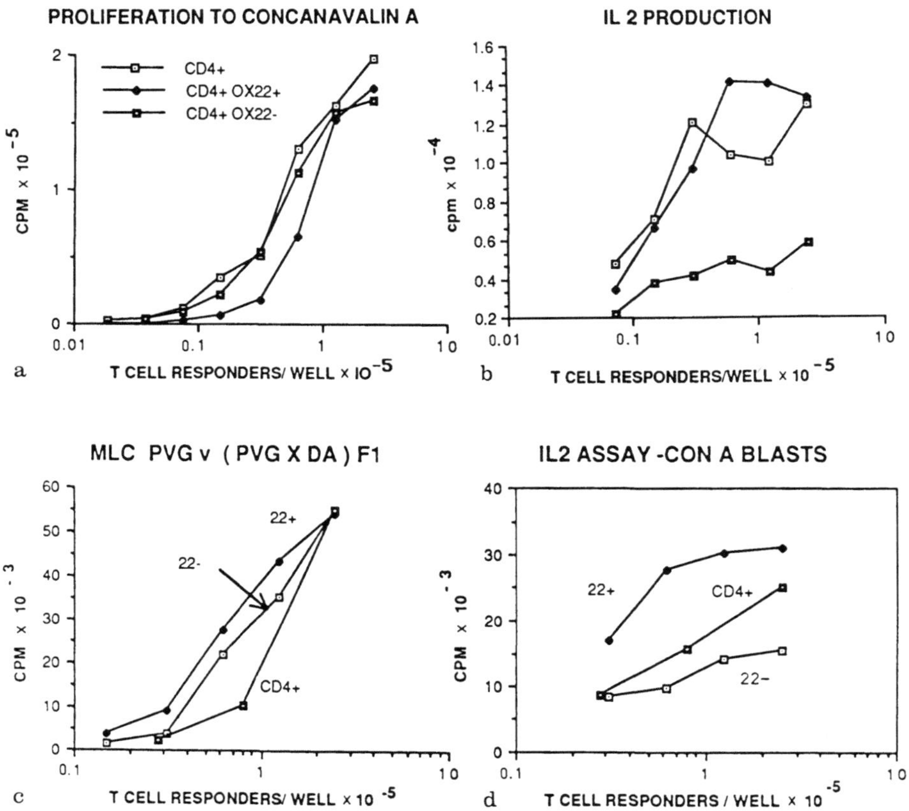


**Fig. 3 a-d.** Proliferative responses of MRC OX-22$^+$ and MRC OX-22$^-$ subsets of CD4$^+$ T cells to Con A (**a**) or alloantigen (**c**) and measurement of concomitant interleukin-2 (*IL-2*) production (**b, d**). CD4$^+$ T cells were isolated from PVG TDL and separated into MRC OX-22$^+$ and MRC OX-22$^-$ fractions as described in (ARTHUR and MASON 1986). The purified subpopulations and unseparated CD4$^+$ T cells were aliquoted in 200-$\mu$l culture volumes of RPMI supplemented with 5% FCS containing 5 $\mu$g/ml Con A and $5 \times 10^5$ T-cell-depleted 2000 R irradiated syngeneic splenocytes (**a**) and $5 \times 10^5$ 2000 R irradiated (PVG × DA) F1 splenocytes (**c**) as stimulator cells. Proliferation was assessed with an 18-h $^3$H-thymidine (0.5 $\mu$Ci) pulse added after 48 h (**a**) or 72 h (**c**) incubation. Supernatants were harvested after 48 h (**a**) or 72 h (**c**) culture and assayed for T-cell growth factor activity using $1 \times 10^4$ cytolytic T lymphocytes (CTLL) as responders (**b**) or $4 \times 10^4$ rat splenic Con A blasts (**d**). Data are means of duplicate determinations. PVG and DA are inbred rat strains with different Major Listocompatibility complex allotypes.

interleukin-2 antagonists (LELCHUK and PLAYFAIR 1985; NELSON and SHNEIDER 1974), and the failure of the OX-22$^-$ CD4$^+$ cells to respond in these proliferation assays when rat serum was present can probably be attributed to the combination of low lymphokine production and the presence of antagonists to it.

Support for this suggestion comes from the finding that the proliferation in fetal calf serum of the OX-22$^-$ CD4$^+$ subset in the MLC can be almost completely inhibited by monoclonal antibody to the rat interleukin-2 receptor[2],

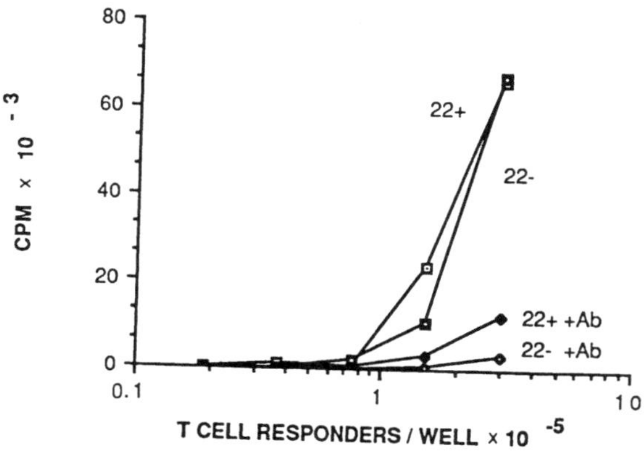


**Fig. 4.** Inhibition of the mixed leucocyte reaction with anti-IL-2 receptor (*R*)mABs. Cells and culture conditions were exactly as described for Fig. 3c except 10 μg/ml NDS-62 (anti-IL-2R mAB) was added to the culture wells. Proliferation was assessed with an 18 h $^3$H-thymidine pulse added after 48 h incubation. Data are means of duplicate determinations. Two further experiments generated similar results. *Ab*, antibody

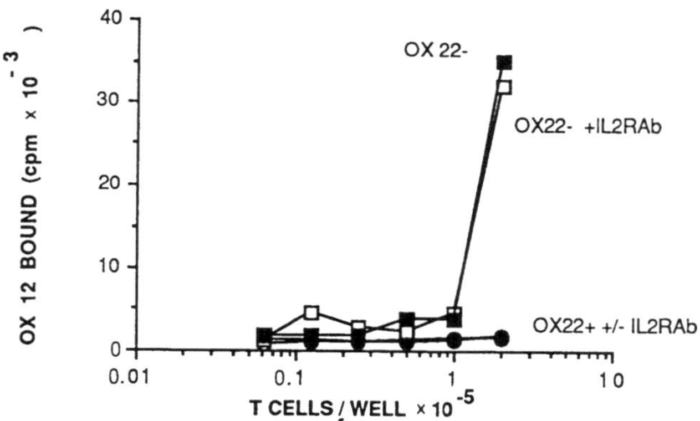


**Fig. 5.** Anti-IL-2R mAb does not prevent OX-22$^-$CD$^+$ cells from providing helper activity for B cells. TDL from rats primed with 0.5 mg DNP-BGG about 6 weeks earlier were separated into OX-22$^+$CD4$^+$ and OX-22$^-$CD4$^+$ fractions as described (Arthur and Mason 1986). The purified subpopulations and unseparated CD4$^+$T cells were aliquoted in duplicate 300 μl culture volumes of RPMI with 10% FCS containing 4 × 10$^5$ primed B cells (obtained by rosette depletion of TDL with anti-CD8 and anti-CD4 mAbs), 5 × 10$^5$ T-cell-depleted, 2000 R irradiated splenic accessory cells and 10 ng DNP-BGG per millilitre in the presence or absence of 10 μg anti-IL-2R mAb per millilitre and cultured for 6 days. Supernatant obtained at this time was assayed for the presence of anti-DNP antibody in a solid phase RIA. All data are the means of duplicate determinations. Control supernatant from cultures containing no T cells gave 2000 cpm bound. A further experiment gave a similar result

whereas less profound inhibition can be obtained when the OX-22$^+$ CD4$^+$ subset is used as the responder population (Fig. 4). The small amounts of interleukin-2 that the OX-22$^-$ CD4$^+$ subset does produce seem to play no essential role in the provision of helper activity for B cells since the inclusion of anti-interleukin-2 receptor antibody, at concentrations that virtually completely inhibit the MLC,

[2] Monoclonal antibody NDS62 is believed to be against the rat interleukin-2 receptor on the basis of the fact that it binds only to activated T cells that are interleukin-2 receptor positive and that it precipitates from these cells a 55-kDa surface antigen. (It was the kind gift of Dr. M. Dallman.)

does not eliminate antibody production by primed B cell co-cultured with primed OX-22$^-$ CD4$^+$ T cells and antigen (Fig. 5).

## 6 Stability of the OX-22$^+$ CD4$^+$ Phenotype

The rat thymus contains only about 2% OX-22$^+$ thymocytes (SPICKETT et al. 1983). Phenotypic analysis of this small population reveals that the majority (> 90%) are CD4$^-$ and CD8$^-$, i.e. they do not have the phenotype of mature peripheral T cells (D. PATERSON, personal communication). It follows that if CD4$^+$ cells become OX-22$^+$ within the thymus they must leave the organ very soon afterwards. Alternatively, peripheral OX-22$^-$ CD4$^+$ cells may contain a population of recent thymic migrants that have yet to express the OX-22 antigen. There is some evidence that this is so since about 50% of peripheral OX-22$^-$ CD4$^+$ T cells express antigen ER-T8[3] (JOLING et al. 1985), which is absent on the majority of rat peripheral T cells but is expressed on all thymocytes (D. MASON, unpublished data). Bearing in mind the hazards of trying to deduce cell lineages from cell phenotypes, this evidence is clearly inconclusive. Regardless of this uncertainty, there is convincing data that the OX-22$^+$ CD4$^+$ phenotype, once acquired, is not stable. The in vitro activation of purified OX-22$^+$ CD4$^+$ T cells by T-cell mitogen results in the generation of CD4$^+$ T-cell blasts that do not express the OX-22 antigen (Table 3). Similarly, CD4$^+$ T-cell lines and clones specific for guinea-pig myelin basic protein also fail to express this determinant (data not shown).

**Table 3.** Loss of expression of the OX-22 epitope on T-cell activation

| Phenotype of starting population | Purity (%) | Positive cells after 8 days in culture (%) OX-21 | IL-2R | OX-40 | OX-22 | CD4 |
|---|---|---|---|---|---|---|
| CD4$^+$ OX-22$^+$ | 98.5 | 21 | 56 | 40 | 26 | 99 |
| Unseparated CD4$^+$ | 99 | 7 | 39 | 29 | 13 | 99 |

CD4$^+$ and separated OX-22$^+$CD4$^+$TDL were set up in culture at $1 \times 10^6$ per millilitre in the presence of 5 $\mu$g ConA per millilitre and $5 \times 10^5$ 2000 R irradiated splenic accessory cells. After 3 days in culture the cells were washed and fresh medium containing 5 $\mu$g Con A per millilitre was added. After a further 2 days the cells were washed again and resuspended in RPMI with 10% FCS. The cells were rested in these culture conditions for 3 days after which viable T cells were isolated by Isopaque Ficoll separation and phenotyped by FACS analysis. The cells recovered had increased tenfold from the starting population. Antibodies used: OX-40 mAb reacts with an antigen found only on activated CD4$^+$ T cells (PATERSON et al. 1987). OX-21 is reactive with the human C3b inactivator and is used here as a reagent control.
Note that the percentage of cells labelled with the OX-22 antibody is only slightly larger than that obtained using OX-21 antibody.

[3] The monoclonal antibody ER-T8 precipitates a 25-kDa antigen from rat thymocytes (JOLING et al. 1985). The ER-T8 used in our experiments was prepared at the Erasmus University, Rotterdam, Netherlands and was the kind gift of Dr. JAN ROSING

**Table 4.** Phenotype of TDL from T-cell-replaced congenitally athymic rats and B rats 8–10 weeks after reconstitution

| Reconstitution | Total TDL output in 18 h | Positive cells (% of the total) | | | | | | |
|---|---|---|---|---|---|---|---|---|
| | | $CD4^+$ | $CD8^+$ | Surface $Ig^+$ | $CD4^+$ $OX\text{-}22^-$ | $CD4^+$ $OX\text{-}22^+$ | $IL\text{-}2R^+$ | $OX\text{-}40^+$ |
| A. Congenitally athymic rats[a] | | | | | | | | |
| $1-5\times10^6$ $CD4^+$ TDL | $1.9\times10^8$ $(1.1-2.7\times10^8)$ | 21 | 2 | 67 | 20 | 2.7 | 10 | 14 |
| $1-5\times10^6$ $CD4^+$ $OX\text{-}22^+$ TDL | $1.4\times10^8$ $(0.6-2.3\times10^8)$ | 48 | 2 | 43 | 45 | 1.3 | 23 | 37 |
| $1-5\times10^6$ $CD4^+$ $OX\text{-}22^-$ TDL | $2.6\times10^8$ $(1.9-3.3\times10^8)$ | 11 | 3 | 79 | 10.5 | 1.6 | 6 | 6 |
| Unreconstituted[c] *rnu/rnu* | $2.3\times10^7$ | 2 | 2 | 83 | 2 | 1 | 0.6 | N.D. |
| Normal PVG | $3\times10^8$ $(2-3.8\times10^8)$ | 39 | 7 | 51 | 14 | 23 | 1 | 1 |
| B. B rats[b] | | | | | | | | |
| $2\times10^6$ $CD4^+$ TDL | $2.0\times10^8$ $(1.0-3.3\times10^8)$ | 25 | 2 | 74 | 21 | 3 | 7 | N.D. |
| $2\times10^6$ $CD4^+$ $OX\text{-}22^+$ TDL | $1.43\times10^8$ $(0.43-1.98\times10^8)$ | 41 | 2 | 56 | 38 | 3 | 12 | 22 |
| $2\times10^6$ $CD4^+$ $0X\text{-}22^-$ TDL | $1.5\times10^8$ $(1.34-1.76\times10^8)$ | 17 | 2 | 82 | 14 | 3 | 3 | 3 |
| Unreconstituted B Rat | $1\times10^8$ $(0.2-2\times10^8)$ | 5 | 1 | 90 | 5 | 1 | 1 | 1 |

[a]Congenitally athymic rats of PVG background were reconstituted with $1-5\times10^6$ fractionated PVG $CD4^+$T cells. After 8–10 weeks the recipients were cannulated and TDL were collected overnight. Numbers in parentheses are the ranges of TDL output which it will be noted are independent of dose of injected T cells. The TDL were phenotyped by indirect two-colour immunofluorescence on a FACS. Data are the mean values of three animals taken from two experiments
[b]Exactly as for A except the recipients were PVG rats rendered T-cell-deficient by thymectomy, two doses of 600 R irradiation over 3 days followed by reconstitution with bone marrow depleted of T cells
[c]n = 1

Comparable results have been obtained in vivo. When congenitally athymic rats, or rats rendered T-cell deficient by thymectomy, lethal irradiation and bone marrow reconstitution (B rats), are injected with syngeneic OX-22$^+$ CD4$^+$ T cells there is extensive expansion of the injected cells, resulting in 100- to 1000-fold expansion in T-cell numbers (Bell et al. 1987; Mason and Simmonds 1988). However, the CD4$^+$ cells recovered after this expansion are OX-22$^-$. That these cells derive from the OX-22$^+$ CD4$^+$ cells in the original inoculum, and not from a very minor contamination with cells of OX-22$^-$ CD4$^+$ phenotype, is supported by the fact that similar T-cell-deficient rats given purified OX-22$^-$ CD4$^+$ T cells reconstitute their T-cell pool less fully (Table 4). These in vivo data indicate that failure to express the OX-22 determinant is not simply a characteristic of activated T cells since some of the OX-22$^-$CD4$^+$T cells found in rats given purified OX-22$^+$CD4$^+$ cells appear to have reverted to a resting state in as much as they do not express interleukin-2 receptors or the OX-40 antigen, a marker for activated CD4$^+$T cells (Paterson et al. 1987). This is more obvious in the reconstitution of the B rats (Table 4b). Finally, there is evidence that CD8$^+$ T cells undergo a similar phenotypic change in that virtually all these cells in TDL from specific pathogen free rats are OX-22$^+$, whereas the CD8$^+$ cytotoxic effector cell does not express the OX-22 antigen (Dallman 1982).

## 7 T Cells that Provide Help for B Cells in Primary Responses Are of the OX-22$^+$ CD4$^+$ Phenotype

When T-cell deficient rats are given syngeneic inocula of either OX-22$^+$ CD4$^+$ or OX-22$^-$CD4$^+$T cells and immunized with ovalbumin or dinitrophenyl-ovalbumin, it is the recipients of the OX-22$^+$ subset that make an anti-ovalbumin or anti-hapten antibody response (Fig. 6). Given that OX-22$^+$ CD4$^+$ cells in such recipients become OX-22$^-$ after injection and that memory helper T cells have the OX-22$^-$ CD4$^+$ phenotype, it seems most probable that these memory cells derive from OX-22$^+$ precursors. The alternative hypothesis, that the memory helper cell derives from a precursor that is itself OX-22$^-$, is not compatible with the fact that no helper activity can be obtained from OX-22$^-$ CD$^+$T cells from unprimed donors. These results and the ones referred to concerning the CD8$^+$T-cell subset suggest the following lineage relationships:

| Thymus → | Periphery → (naive cells) | Pheriphery → (activated cells) | Periphery (memory cells) |
|---|---|---|---|
| OX-22$^-$CD4$^+$ | OX-22$^+$CD4$^+$ | OX-22$^-$CD4$^+$ | OX-22$^-$CD4$^+$ |
| OX-22$^-$CD8$^+$ | OX-22$^+$CD8$^+$ | OX-22$^-$CD8$^+$ | OX-22$^-$CD8$^+$ |

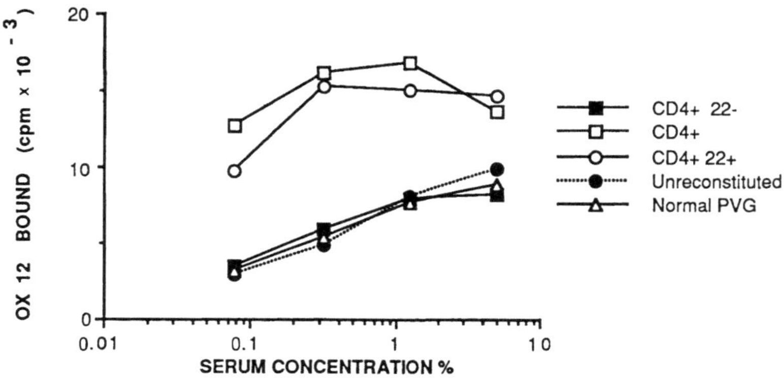


**Fig. 6.** T cells that provide help for B cells in primary responses are of the OX-22$^+$CD4$^+$ phenotype. Nude rats were given $5 \times 10^6$ OX-22$^+$CD4$^+$ ($n = 3$), $5 \times 10^6$ CD4$^+$ ($n = 3$) or $1.5 \times 10^6$ 22$^-$CD4$^+$ ($n = 2$) T cells separated from normal PVG TDL. Two animals were unreconstituted. At this time the animals were immunized with an alum precipitate of 0.5 mg DNP-ovalbumin and $10^9$ pertussis organisms intraperitoneally. The data represent the mean anti-DNP antibody response in the sera of these animals at day 14, as assessed by solid-phase RIA (SPICKETT et al. 1983). The range of the data is not shown as it was less than 5% of the mean value for all points. A further experiment using B rats reconstituted with CD4$^+$ T-cell subpopulations and immunized with 100 μg ovalbumin gave similar results. In this experiment all animals received the same T-cell dose ($2 \times 10^6$ cells)

# 8 The Problem with Interleukin-2-Producing Cells

The above sequence, while supported by the data on the helper activity of T cells for primary and secondary antibody responses, does raise difficulties with respect to cells that produce interleukin-2. As noted, interleukin-2 production by OX-22$^-$CD4$^+$T cells is poor in comparison with that from cells with the OX-22$^+$ phenotype even when the former cells are responding vigorously to the non-specific mitogen Con A. It seems that cells of memory phenotype do not simply correspond to a homogeneous expansion of naive cells. A similar conclusion is suggested by the finding that in man 2H4$^+$CD4$^+$T cells can induce suppression by CD8$^+$T cells of pokeweed mitogen-driven immunoglobulin production by B cells, but the 2H4$^-$ T cells cannot (MORIMOTO et al. 1985). A number of explanations for these results can be advanced. It has been suggested for example, with regard to the human data, that 2H4$^+$ suppressor-inducer T cells undergo further differentiation to become 2H4$^-$ helper cells for secondary antibody responses (BEVERLY 1986/87). Studies on T-cell clones in the mouse are relevant here and have shown that they fall into two non-overlapping groups: those that make interleukin-2 and those that make interleukin-4 (CHERWINSKI et al. 1987; KILLAR et al. 1987). Since interleukin-4 plays a major role in B-cell proliferation and differentiation (KILLAR et al. 1987; BOOM et al. 1988), it is apparent that the clones producing this lymphokine resemble more closely OX-22$^-$CD$^+$T cell, while precursors of clones that produce interleukin-2 would appear to be represented predominantly in the OX-22$^+$CD4$^+$ subset. Significantly, no mouse

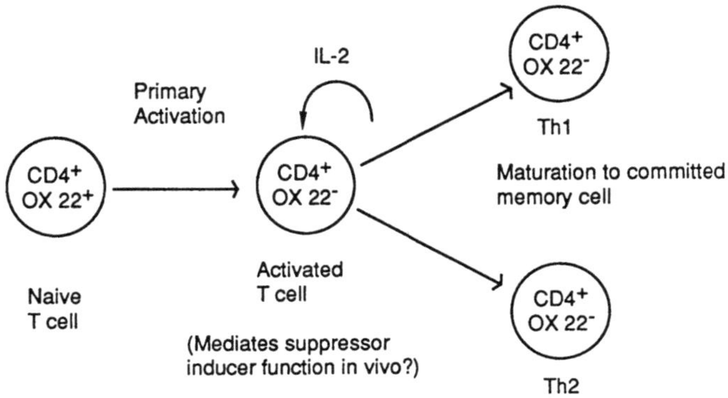


**Fig. 7.** Possible maturation sequence of $CD4^+$ T cells

T-cell clone has been found that has switched its lymphokine production, suggesting that once T cells have reached the level of differentiation represented by these clones the repertoire of lymphokine production is stable. If a similar situation applied to the two subsets of rat $CD4^+$ cells then it could be concluded that $OX\text{-}22^+CD4^+$T cells that produce interleukin-2 on primary activation do not go on to become memory cells that help B cells in secondary antibody responses. Similar considerations could be applied to the corresponding human T-cell subsets. However, bearing in mind that the primary activation of T cells in vivo probably required that they encounter antigen presented by specialised dendritic cells (Inaba and Steinman 1984) found in the T areas of lymph nodes and spleen, it may be that in these regions naive $CD4^+$T cells undergo clonal expansion mediated by the autocrine action of interleukin-2 (Smith 1984) and that their progeny then become committed to the production of a particular lymphokine repertoire corresponding to one or other of the two types of mouse T-cell clone (Fig. 7). A precedent for this type of bidirectional differentiation can be found in other leucocytes, for example where granulocytes and macrophages develop as a mixed colony from the clonal expansion of a common precursor (Metcalf 1984). Final resolution of the problem of IL-2 production by subsets of rat $CD4^+$ T cells must await the development of a monoclonal antibody that, like 2H4 antibody in man (Mason and Powrie, submitted), splits the $OX\text{-}22^+$ $CD4^+$ subset into naive and memory T cell fractions.

## 9 Interactions In Vivo Between Subsets of $CD4^+$ T Cells

As already described, congenitally athymic rats given $1-5 \times 10^6$ $CD4^+$ T cells of either $OX\text{-}22^+$ or $OX\text{-}22^-$ phenotype are found to have large numbers of $OX\text{-}22^-$ $CD4^+$ T cells in their thoracic duct lymph within 8 weeks of cell injection

(Table 4A). Despite the similar proliferative capacity of the two $CD4^+$ subsets, the OX-22 phenotype of the $CD4^+$ T cells injected has a profound effect on the subsequent fate of the recipient rats. Animals given unfractionated $CD4^+$ T cells or those given the $OX\text{-}22^-CD4^+$ subset continue to thrive, whereas recipients of $OX\text{-}22^+CD4^+$ cells invariably become severely wasted and, unless culled, finally succumb, having lost at least 50% of their body weight. As Table 4A shows, such wasted animals contain a very much higher frequency of $CD4^+$ T cells that express interleukin-2 receptors and the activation marker OX-40 than do recipients of either unseparated $CD4^+$ T cells or the $OX\text{-}22^-$ subset thereof. As rats given unfractionated $CD4^+$ T cells receive $OX\text{-}22^+CD4^+$ cells but remain healthy, it appears that the concomitant transfer of the $OX\text{-}22^-CD4^+$ subset both prevents the wasting disease that $OX\text{-}22^+CD4^+$ T cells alone induce and moderates their activation. At present the cause of the wasting disease is not understood, nor is it known how the $OX\text{-}22^-CD4^+$ T cells prevent it. One possibility is that this subset is involved in suppressing autoreactivity as there is evidence that rats contain potentially autoaggressive T cells that are actively held in check (BELLGRAU et al. 1981). However, other explanations can be advanced and further work is indicated to help resolve the alternatives.

There is also some evidence for a reciprocal regulating mechanism in that congenitally athymic rats given $OX\text{-}22^-CD4^+$ T cells are found to have a very high frequency of B cells in their thoracic duct lymph compared with euthymic animals. This B-cell expansion is not evident in the animals given the $22^+$ subset of $CD4^+$ T cells (Table 4A).

Recalling that $2H4^+CD4^+$ T cells in man can induce suppression of B-cell activation by pokeweed mitogen (MORIMOTO et al. 1985), it is tempting to suggest that $OX\text{-}22^+CD4^+$ T cells in vivo play an analogous role. In any event, the in vivo data taken together do suggest that $OX\text{-}22^+CD4^+$ T cells do not simply serve as precursors of $OX\text{-}22^-$ cells that mediate immune responses solely to environmental antigens, and the true situation appears to be more dynamic than this rather pastoral view portrays.

## 10 The Function of the CD45 Molecule

The CD45 molecule is uncommon among leukocyte membrane molecules studied so far in that it has such a large cytoplasmic part and it is notable that the amino acid sequence of this portion of CD45 is more highly conserved in phylogeny than is the remainder of the molecule (RALPH et al. 1987). Recent work (TONKS et al. 1988) has shown that this portion of the molecule has protein tyrosine phosphatase activity and is involved in leucocyte activation (PINGEL and THOMAS 1989).

The extracellular part of the CD45 molecule is heavily glycosylated in the $NH_2$-terminal region where variation in sequence due to differential RNA splicing is found. It is possible that this region makes low-affinity interactions with lectin-like molecules on other cells or connective tissue elements (THOMAS et al. 1987). If this is the case then the various forms of CD45 presumably allow specific interactions to occur that depend on the particular forms of CD45 expressed. Given the demonstrable role of this molecules in the activation of a variety of cell types (SPARROW and MCKENZIE 1983; VAKURA et al. 1983; HARP et al. 1984; TAKEUCHI et al. 1987; PINGEL and THOMAS 1989) it is possible that the interaction of the extracellular portion of CD45 with its specific ligands plays a crucial role in determining whether cell activation takes place of not, even in those situations where the other conditions for activation, such as the engagement of T- or B-cell antigen receptors with their appropriately presented target molecules, are met. If this hypothesis is correct then one may envisage that the various isoforms of the CD45 molecule on different T cell subsets determine which type of antigen-presenting cells can lead to T cell activation or in which anatomical locations such activation can take place.

*Acknowledgements.* Our thanks are due to Steve Simmonds for expert technical assistance, to Reg Boone for running the cell sorter, to Stan Buckingham for prompt photographic service and to Allison Thomas for secretarial help. Fiona Powrie is in receipt of an Arthritis and Rheumatism Council research studentship.

## References

Arthur RP, Mason D (1986) T cells that help B cell responses to soluble antigen are distinguishable from those producing interleukin 2 on mitogenic or allogeneic stimulation. J Exp Med 163: 774–786

Barclay AN, Jackson DI, Willis AC, Williams AF (1987) Lymphocyte specific heterogeneity in the rat leucocyte common antigen (T200) is due to differences in polypeptide sequence near the $NH_2$-terminus. EMBO J 6: 1259–1264

Bell EB, Sparshott SM, Drayson MT, Ford WL (1987) The stable and permanent expansion of functional T lymphocytes in athymic nude rats after a single injection of mature T cells. J Immunol 139: 1379–1384

Bellgrau D, Smilik D, Wilson DB (1981) Induced tolerance in F1 rats to anti-major histocompatibility complex receptors on parental T cells. J Exp Med 153: 1660–1665

Beverley PCL (1986/87) Human T cell subsets. Immunol Lett 14: 263–267

Boom WH, Liano D, Abbas AK (1988) Heterogeneity of helper/inducer T lymphocytes II. Effects of interleukin-4 and interleukin 2-producing T cell clones on resting B lymphocytes. J Exp Med 167: 1350–1363

Cantor H, Boyse EA (1975) Functional subclasses of T lymphocytes bearing different Ly antigens. II. Cooperation between subclasses of $Ly^+$ cells in the generation of killer activity. J Exp Med 141: 1390–1399

Cherwinski H, Schumacher JH, Brown KD, Mossman TR (1987) Two types of mouse helper T cell clone. III. Further differences in lymphokine synthesis between Th1 and Th2 clones revealed by RNA hybridization, functionally monospecific bioassays and monoclonal antibodies. J Exp Med 166: 1229–1244

Cobbold S, Hale G, Waldmann H (1987) Non lineage, LFA-1 family and leukocyte common antigens: new and previously defined clusters. In: McMichael AJ (ed) Leukocyte typing III. Oxford University Press, Oxford, pp 788–807

Dalchau R, Kirkley J, Fabre JW (1980) Monoclonal antibody to a human leukocyte specific membrane glycoprotein probably homologous to the leukocyte-common (L-C) antigen of the rat. Eur J Immunol 10: 737–744

Dallman MJ (1982) Studies on the cellular basis of skin allograft rejection in the rat. D Phil thesis, Oxford

Fabre JW, Williams AF (1977) Quantitative serological analysis of a rabbit anti-rat lymphocyte serum and preliminary biochemical characterization of the major antigen recognised. Transplantation 23: 349–359

Ford WL, Burr W, Simonsen M (1970) A lymph node weight assay for the graft-versus-host reactivity of rat lymphoid cells. Transplantation 10: 258–266

Harp JA, Davis BS, Ewald SJ (1984) Inhibition of T cell responses to alloantigens and polyclonal mitogens by Ly-5 antisera. J Immunol 133: 10–15

Inaba K, Steinman RM (1984) Resting and sensitized T lymphocytes exhibit distinct stimulatory (antigen-presenting cell) requirements for growth and lymphokine release. J Exp Med 160: 1717–1735

Joling P, Tielen FJ, Vaessen LMB, Huijbregts JMA, Rozing J (1985) New markers on T cell subpopulations defined by monoclonal antibodies. Transplant Proc 17: 1857–1863

Killar L, MacDonald G, West J, Woods A, Bottomly K (1987) Cloned, Ia-restricted T cells that do not produce interleukin 4 (IL4)/B cell stimulatory factor 1 (BSF-1) fail to help antigen-specific B cells. J Immunol 138: 1674–1679

Lelchuk R, Playfair JHL (1985) Serum IL-2 inhibitor in mice. I. Increase during infection. Immunology 56: 113–118

Mason DW, Simmonds SJ (1988) The autonomy of CD8$^+$ T cell in vitro and in vivo. Immunology 65: 249–257

Mason DW, Brideau RJ, McMaster WR, Webb M, White RAH, Williams AF (1980) Monoclonal antibodies that define T-lymphocyte subsets in the rat. In: Kennett RH, McKern TJ, Bechtol KB (eds) Monoclonal antibodies. Plenum, New York, pp 251–273

Mason DW, Penhale WJ, Sedgwick JD (1987) Preparation of lymphocyte subpopulations. In: Klaus GGB (ed) Lymphocytes, a practical approach. IRL Press, Oxford, pp 35–54

Metcalf D (1984) The hemopoietic colony stimulating factors. Elsevier, Amsterdam, p 33

Morimoto C, Letvin NL, Distaso JA, Aldrich WR, Schlossman SF (1985) The isolation and characterization of the human suppressor inducer T cell subset. J Immunol 134: 1508–1515

Nelson DS, Sneider C (1974) Effect of normal mouse serum on mouse lymphocyte transformation in vitro. Eur J Immunol 4: 79–86

Paterson DJ, Jefferies WA, Green JR, Brandon MR, Corthesy P, Puklavec M, Williams AF (1987) Antigens of activated rat T lymphocytes including a molecule of 50 000 $M_r$ detected only on CD4 positive T blasts. Mol Immunol 24: 1281–1290

Pingel JR, Thomas ML (1989) Evidence that the leukocyte-common antigen is required for antigen-induced T lymphocyte proliferation. Cell 58: 1055–1065

Ralph SJ, Thomas ML, Morton CC, Trowbridge IS (1987) Structural variants of human T200 glycoprotein (leukocyte-common antigen). EMBO J 6: 1251–1257

Reinherz, EL, Schlossman SF (1980) The differentiation and function of human T lymphocytes. A review. Cell 19: 821–827

Saga Y, Tung JS, Shen FW, Boyse EA (1987) Alternative use of 5′ exons in the specification of Ly-5 isoforms distinguishing hematopoietic cell lineages. Proc Natl Acad Sci USA 84: 5364–5368

Smith KA (1984) Interleukin 2. Annu Rev Immunol 2: 319–333

Sparrow RL, McKenzie IFC (1983) A function for human T200 in natural killer cytolysis. Transplantation 36: 166–171

Spickett GP, Brandon MR, Mason DW, Williams AF, Woollett GR (1983) MRC OX-22, a monoclonal antibody that labels a new subset of T lymphocytes and reacts with the high molecular weight form of the leukocyte-common antigen. J Exp Med 158: 795–810

Standring R, McMaster WR, Sunderland CA, Williams AF (1978) The predominant heavily glycosylated glycoproteins at the surface of rat lymphoid cells are differentiation antigens. Eur J Immunol 8: 832–839

Streuli M, Hall LR, Saga Y, Schlossman SF, Saito H (1987a) Differential usage of three exons generates at least five different mRNAs encoding human leukocyte common antigens. J Exp Med 166: 1548–1566

Streuli M, Matsuyama T, Morimoto C, Schlossman SF, Saito H (1987b) Identification of the sequence required for expression of the 2H4 epitope on the human leukocyte common antigens. J Exp Med 166: 1567–1572

Streuli M, Morimoto C, Schrieber M, Schlossman SF, Saito H (1988) Characterization of CD45 and CD45R monoclonal antibodies using transfected mouse cell lines that express individual leukocyte-common antigens. J Immunol 141: 3910–3914

Takeuchi T, Rudd CE, Schlossman SF, Morimoto C (1987) Induction of suppression following autologous mixed lymphocyte reaction; role of a novel 2H4 antigen. Eur J Immunol 17: 97–103

Terry LA, Brown MH, Beverley PCL (1988) The monoclonal antibody UCHLI, recognises a 180 000 MW component of the human leukocyte-common antigen, CD45. Immunology 64: 331–336

Thomas ML, Barclay AN, Gagnon J, Williams AF (1985) Evidence from cDNA clones that the rat leukocyte common antigen (T200) spans the lipid bilayer and contains a cytoplasmic domain of 80 000 $M_r$. Cell 41: 83–93

Thomas ML, Reynolds PJ, Chain A, Ben-Neriah Y, Trowbridge IS (1987) B-cell variant of mouse T200 (Ly-5): evidence for alternative in RNA splicing. Proc Natl Acad Sci USA 84: 5360–5363

Tonks NK, Charbonneau H, Diltz CD, Fischer EH, Walsh KA (1988) Demonstration that the leukocyte common antigen CD45 is a protein tyrosine phosphatase. Biochem 27: 8695–8701

Trowbridge IS (1978) Interspecies spleen-myeloma hybrid producing monoclonal antibodies against mouse lymphocyte surface glycoprotein, T200. J Exp Med 148: 313–322

Trowbridge IS, Nilsen-Hamilton M, Hamilton RT, Bevan MJ (1977) Preliminary characterization of two thymus-dependent xenoantigens from mouse lymphocytes. Biochem J 163: 211–217

Williams AF, Galfré G, Milstein C (1977) Analysis of cell surfaces by xenogeneic myeloma-hybrid antibodies: differentiation antigens of rat lymphocytes. Cell 12: 663–673

Woollett GR, Barclay AN, Puklavec M, Williams AF (1985) Molecular and antigenic heterogeneity of the rat leucocyte-common antigen from thymocytes and T and B lymphocytes. Eur J Immunol 15: 168–173

Yakura H, Shen FW, Bourcet E, Boyse EA (1983) On the function of Ly-5 in the regulation of antigen-driven B cell differentiation. Comparison and contrast with Lyb-2. J Exp Med 157: 1077–1088

# Pgp-1 (Ly 24) As a Marker of Murine Memory T Lymphocytes

H. R. MacDonald, R. C. Budd*, and J.-C. Cerottini



## 1 Introduction

It is generally accepted that the primary immune response to an antigen involves the formation of long-lived, antigen-specific memory cells, in addition to effector cells. These memory cells are thought to be responsible for the heightened immune response that follows secondary exposure to an antigen. As the secondary antibody response is generally characterized by the production of increased levels of antibodies having higher avidity for antigen (Eisen and Siskind 1964), it has been proposed that immunologic memory at the B-cell level includes both an increased frequency of antigen-reactive lymphocytes and a greater mean avidity of their antigen receptors (Andersson 1970; Celada 1971; Davie and Paul 1972). In the case of T-cell responses, little is known about the formation of memory cells during immunization. There is evidence that the frequency of antigen-specific T lymphocytes may increase after immunization (MacDonald et al. 1980). In addition, indirect evidence has been provided

Ludwig Institute for Cancer Research, Lausanne Branch, 1066 Epalinges, Switzerland
*Present Address: Genentech Incorporated, San Francisco, California, United States

Current Topics in Microbiology and Immunology, Vol. 159

showing that T cells in immunized animals bear higher avidity antigen receptors compared with normal animals (MACDONALD et al. 1982; MARRACK et al. 1983). However, detailed analysis of memory T cells has been hampered by the lack of suitable surface markers allowing identification and isolation of these cells. As discussed below, recent studies from our laboratory indicate that murine memory T cells can be identified phenotypically by the surface marker Pgp-1. A more comprehensive review of T-cell memory will be presented elsewhere (CEROTTINI and MACDONALD 1989).

## 2 Expression of the Pgp-1 (Ly24) Antigen by T-Lineage Cells

Pgp-1 was originally described (HUGHES et al. 1981, 1983) as a major cell membrane glycoprotein on cultured murine fibroblasts and peritoneal phagocytic cells (hence its designation phagocyte glycoprotein 1). Also designated Ly24, Pgp-1 has a $M_r$ of 80 000–95 000 and is encoded by a locus on chromosome 2 (COLOMBATTI et al. 1982). It has been identified in a wide variety of tissues including brain, liver, kidney, and lung (TROWBRIDGE et al. 1982). In hematopoietic tissues, Pgp-1 is found in highest amounts in the bone marrow. While it is expressed in most prothymocytes (LESLEY et al. 1985a), only about 5% of adult thymocytes are Pgp-1$^+$ The vast majority of these Pgp-1$^+$ thymocytes are confined to the minor ($CD4^-CD8^-$) subset known to contain immature

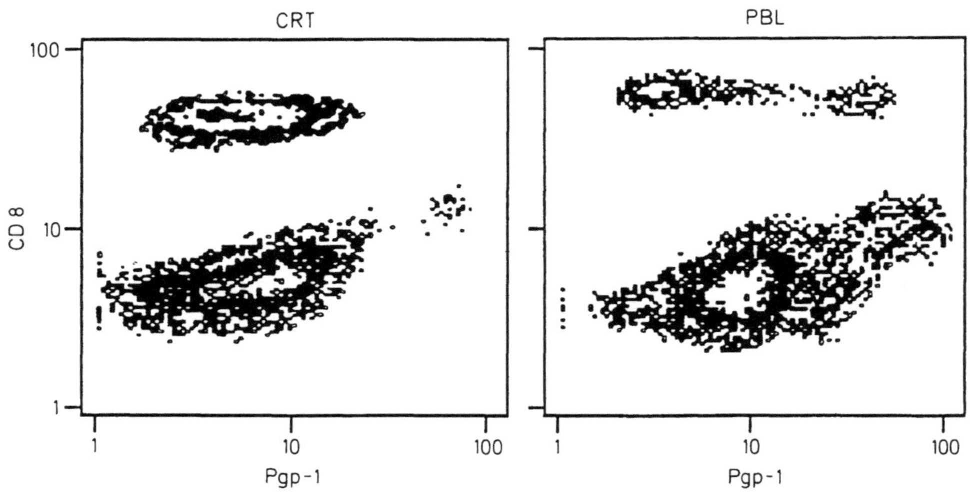


**Fig. 1.** Heterogeneous expression of Pgp-1 by CD8$^+$ T lymphocytes cortisone-resistant thymocytes (CRT) and peripheral blood lymphocytes (PBL) from C57BL/6 mice were double stained with mAbs directed against Pgp-1 (IM 7.8.1; TROWBRIDGE et al. 1982) and CD8 (H-35-17.2; GOLSTEIN et al. 1982). Samples were run on a FACS II flow cytometer with logarithmic fluorescence amplification. Cytogram represents $5 \times 10^4$ viable cells (for technical details see BUDD et al. 1987b)

**Table 1.** Frequency of Pgp-1$^+$ and Pgp-1$^-$ T cells among CD4$^+$ and CD8$^+$ subsets of adult C57BL/6 mice

| Tissue | CD4$^+$ | | CD8$^+$ | |
|---|---|---|---|---|
| | Pgp-1$^-$ | Pgp-1$^+$ | Pgp-1$^-$ | Pgp-1$^+$ |
| Spleen | 71 | 29 | 62 | 38 |
| Lymph node | 88 | 12 | 71 | 29 |
| Peripheral blood | ND | ND | 60 | 40 |
| Thymus[a] | 95 | 5 | 97 | 3 |

Data (mean values of several determinations) were obtained by flow microfluorometry (cf. Fig. 1)
[a]Thymus data refer only to mature (CD4$^+$ CD8$^-$ and CD4$^-$ CD8$^+$) subsets
ND, not done

thymocytes (TROWBRIDGE et al. 1985). Unlike adult thymocytes, the great majority of fetal thymocytes are Pgp-1$^+$ at day 13–14 of gestation (LESLEY et al. 1985b). Thereafter, the proportion of Pgp-1$^+$ thymocytes declines, reaching adult levels by day 19 of gestation. On the basis of these findings, it has been proposed that at least some of the Pgp-1$^+$ cells within the thymus are progenitors of mature thymocytes (LESLEY et al. 1985b).

In contrast to mature (CD8$^+$ and CD4$^+$) thymocytes, peripheral T cells contain a significant proportion of Pgp-1$^+$ cells (BUDD et al. 1987a, b; LYNCH et al. 1987). Figure 1 shows a comparison of Pgp-1 expression by CD8$^+$ cells from cortisone-resistant thymocytes (which are representative of mature thymocytes) and from peripheral blood of C57BL/6 mice. It can be seen that CD8$^+$ blood lymphocytes are separated by Pgp-1 into well-defined dull (Pgp-1$^-$) and bright (Pgp-1$^+$) subpopulations, whereas the vast majority of cortisone-resistant CD8$^+$ thymocytes are Pgp-1$^-$. In the example shown in Fig. 1, 40% of CD8$^+$ blood lymphocytes are Pgp-1$^+$, as compared with only 5% of cortisone-resistant CD8$^+$ thymocytes. In peripheral lymphoid organs, Pgp-1 expression by CD4$^+$ or CD8$^+$ cells is also heterogeneous (Table 1). It should be noted, however, that expression of Pgp-1 does not clearly delineate T-cell subsets in all mouse strains (LYNCH and CEREDIG 1988). Although the basis for this discrepancy is not clear, there is some recent evidence that it is correlated with polymorphism at the Pgp-1 locus (LESLEY et al. 1988).

# 3 Functional Properties of Pgp-1$^+$ T Cells

## 3.1 Size and Cell Cycle Status

Activated lymphocytes undergo blastogenesis and enter the DNA synthesis (S) phase of the cell cycle following stimulation by antigens or mitogenic lectins. A comparison of Pgp-1$^+$ and Pgp-1$^-$ subsets of CD8$^+$ T cells (BUDD et al. 1987b) indicates an increased proportion of blast cells (10%–20%) in the Pgp-1$^+$ fraction; however, no corresponding increase in cycling cells (as assessed by the DNA-binding dye propidium iodide) could be detected. These data indicate that Pgp-1 is not a marker for cycling or activated cells per se; however, the presence of a significant fraction of blasts among Pgp-1$^+$ T cells may reflect an enrichment of recently activated cells in the Pgp-1$^+$ subset (see below).

## 3.2 Antigen-Specific Cytolytic Activity

More direct evidence that Pgp-1 identifies recently activated T cells was obtained by examining the cytolytic activity of peritoneal exudate lymphocytes (PEL) from mice undergoing rejection of an intraperitoneal tumor allograft. In this system, CD8$^+$ Pgp-1$^+$ cells were highly cytolytic against tumor target cells bearing the appropriate major histocompatibility complex (MHC) antigens (50% lysis with an effector to target ratio of 2:1) whereas CD8$^+$ Pgp-1$^-$ cells were noncytolytic (10% lysis at 10:1 ratio; Budd et al. 1987b). Since PEL represent a relatively homogeneous noncycling population of small lymphocytes (Cerottini and Brunner 1974; Berke et al. 1972), these data again suggest that Pgp-1 identifies activated T cells independent of the usual criteria of blast transformation and DNA synthesis.

## 3.3 Frequency of Antigen-Specific Precursor T Cells

Antigen-specific precursor cell frequencies can be determined by limiting dilution analysis, given that the culture conditions utilized are limiting only for the relevant precursor cell (MacDonald et al. 1980). Using this approach, the Pgp-1$^+$ population has been found to contain an enhanced frequency of CD8$^+$ and CD4$^+$ precursor cells specific for a variety of different antigens (Budd et al. 1987a, b; Butterfield et al. 1989). Data from our own studies in mice are summarized in Table 2. It can be seen that CD8$^+$ precursors specific for MHC as

**Table 2.** Enhanced frequency of antigen-specific precursor cells in Pgp-1$^+$ subset of immune mice

| Antigen | Subset | Precursor frequency (reciprocal) | |
|---|---|---|---|
| | | Pgp-1$^-$ | Pgp-1$^+$ |
| Allo-MHC | CD8$^+$ | 30; 20 | 7; 7 |
| Male (H-Y) | CD8$^+$ | 10331 | 341 |
| Virus (MSV) | CD8$^+$ | 626; 1692 | 84; 201 |
| Protein (KLH) | CD4$^+$ | 17400 | 1100 |
| Protein (SWM) | CD4$^+$ | >40000 | 3750 |

Precursor frequencies were measured by limiting dilution analysis. Data are from Budd et al. (1987a, b) and Butterfield et al. (1989). Independent experiments are separated by a semicolon. KLH, keyhole limpet hemocyanin; SWM, sperm whale myoglobin well as minor (H-Y) and viral (murine sarcoma virus) antigens are enriched 3- to 30-fold in the Pgp-1$^+$ subset following immunization in vivo with the appropriate antigen. Data pertaining to CD4$^+$ T cells are more limited at present; however, responses to soluble antigens such as keyhole limpet hemocyanin and sperm whale myoglobin (Table 2), as well as to the intracellular parasite *Leishmania Major* (H. MOLL 1988, personal communication) seem also to involve enrichment of antigen-specific precursor cells in the Pgp-1$^+$ CD4$^+$ subset.

It should be noted that limiting dilution assays detect antigen-specific T cells at all stages of activation including unprimed precursors, functionally active effector cells, and memory cells (MACDONALD et al. 1980). Thus, the frequency differences observed between Pgp-1$^-$ and Pgp-1$^+$ subsets could represent an absolute increase in the number of antigen-specific Pgp-1$^+$ cells (via proliferation) and/or a transition of precursor cells from the Pgp-1$^-$ to the Pgp-1$^+$ compartment. These possibilities will be discussed in detail in a later section.

## 3.4 Production of Lymphokines

T lymphocytes secrete a bewildering variety of soluble mediators (referred to collectively as lymphokines) following antigenic or mitogenic stimulation. It has been known for some time that T cells from immunized animals produce larger amounts of certain lymphokines than unprimed T cells; however, it has been difficult to distinguish whether this increased production can be accounted for solely by an increased frequency of antigen-specific precursor cells following immunization. As shown in Table 3, Pgp-1$^+$ cells of both the CD4$^+$ and CD8$^+$ subsets produce greater amounts of the lymphokines IFN-$\gamma$ and (to a lesser extent) interleukin-3 (IL-3) than Pgp-1$^-$ cells when stimulated with mitogens. Parallel results have been obtained for IL-4 (T. MOSMANN and R.C. BUDD 1988, personal communication). In contrast, IL-2 production is comparable in the Pgp-1$^+$ and Pgp-1$^-$ subsets. Taken together with similar results in man (SANDERS et al. 1988), our data suggest strongly that Pgp-1$^+$ T cells (on a per cell basis) secrete more of certain lymphokines than their Pgp-1$^-$ counterparts. Furthermore, they raise the possibility that regulation of expression of the IFN-$\gamma$ and

**Table 3.** Lymphokine production by Pgp-1$^-$ and Pgp-1$^+$ T-cell subsets

| Lymphokine | CD4$^+$ | | CD8$^+$ | |
|---|---|---|---|---|
| | Pgp-1$^-$ | Pgp-1$^+$ | Pgp-1$^-$ | Pgp-1$^+$ |
| IL-2 | 120[a] | 125 | 270 | 330 |
| IL-3 | 11 | 80 | <5 | 57 |
| IFN-$\gamma$ | <5 | 170 | 7 | 130 |

Data are for a representative experiment in which cells were stimulated with phorbol myristate acetate (10 ng/ml) plus ionomycin (500 ng/ml) for 24 h. For complete data see BUDD et al. (1987c)

[a]Reciprocal of supernatant titer yielding 50% maximal acitivity

IL-4 genes can be controlled independently of the expression of other lymphokine genes such as IL-2 (see TANIGUCHI 1988).

Recent studies in several laboratories have drawn attention to the fact that long-term T-cell clones of the $CD4^+$ phenotype can be divided into two categories ($T_H1$ and $T_H2$) based on their pattern of lymphokine secretion (MOSMANN and COFFMAN 1987). This compartmentalization seems unlikely to correlate with expression of Pgp-1, since two lymphokine activities that are increased among $CD4^+$ Pgp-$1^+$ cells (IL-4 and IFN-$\gamma$) are expressed by mutually exclusive subsets of long-term T-cell clones.

## 3.5 Affinity of T-Cell Receptors

T-cell antigen receptors (TCR) consist of a variable $\alpha/\beta$ heterodimer non-covalenty associated with a nonpolymorphic complex referred to as CD3. As mentioned previously, maturation of B lymphocytes in vivo is accompanied by an increase in the affinity of the antibodies they secrete. In the case of T lymphocytes, receptor affinities cannot be measured directly since the TCR complex reacts with a poorly defined complex of MHC molecule and peptide antigen on the stimulator cell surface. However, relative affinities of TCR can be indirectly compared by varying the concentration of antigen/MHC complex on the stimulator cell (MARRACK et al. 1983; SHIMONKEVITZ et al. 1985) or by neutralizing the avidity-enhancing function of accessory molecules such as CD4 and CD8 (MACDONALD et al. 1982; SWAIN 1983). From this type of analysis, there is evidence that immunization in vivo selects for antigen-specific TCR of relatively higher affinity than the majority of those TCR expressed by unprimed T cells (MACDONALD et al. 1982).

When alloimmune $CD8^+$ T cells were sorted into Pgp-$1^-$ and Pgp-$1^+$ subsets

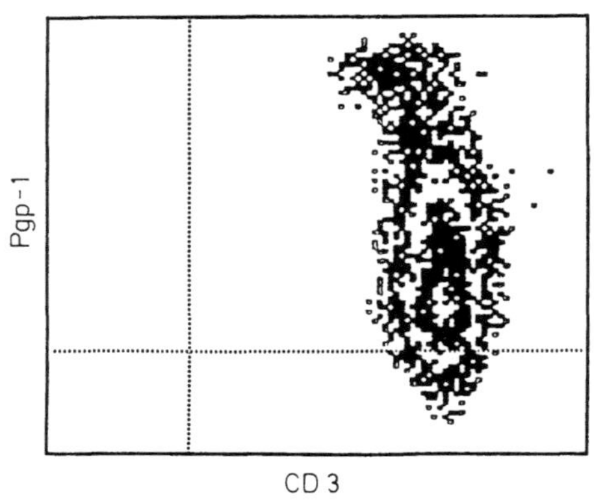


**Fig. 2.** CD3 expression by Pgp-$1^+$ and Pgp-$1^-$ subsets of $CD8^+$ T lymphocytes. CD4-depleted nylon wool purified lymph node cells from C57BL/6 mice were double stained with mAbs directed against CD3 (145-2C11; LEO et al. 1987) and Pgp-1 (IM 7.8.1). Samples were analyzed as in Fig. 1. The *dotted lines* represent the means of controls stained with the fluorescent conjugates alone. Independent staining established that all $CD3^+$ cells were $CD8^+$ (not shown)

and plated at limiting dilution, cytolysis mediated by the resulting Pgp-1$^+$ "clones" was found to be much more resistant to inhibition by anti-CD8 monoclonal antibodies (mAbs) than was the case for the corresponding Pgp-1$^-$ "clones" (BUDD et al. 1987a). This was not the case in unprimed mice, where both Pgp-1$^+$ and Pgp-1$^-$ subsets gave rise to "clones" that were equally susceptible to anti-CD8 inhibition. Taken together with earlier studies (MACDONALD et al. 1982), these data suggest that the Pgp-1$^+$ subset in immune animals is enriched with respect to antigen-specific T cells bearing high-affinity TCR. Evidence that the affinity (rather than density) of TCR accounts for this difference comes from the observation that CD3 staining (and hence presumably TCR density) is not significantly different in the Pgp-1$^+$ and Pgp-1$^-$ subset of CD8$^+$ T cells (Fig. 2).

## 3.6 Growth Requirements In Vitro

In initial studies, we observed that Pgp-1$^+$ and Pgp-1$^-$ subsets of both CD4$^+$ and CD8$^+$ T lymphocytes proliferated equivalently when stimulated by the combination of phorbol ester and calcium ionophore (BUDD et al. 1987c). As shown recently by others (SCHMIDBERGER et al. 1988; MIETHKE et al. 1988), immobilized anti-CD3 mAbs are a convenient (and perhaps more physiological) tool with which to study the activation and growth of murine T cells following TCR triggering. By applying this system to sorted CD8$^+$ T cells plated at low cell density, we have found that both Pgp-1$^+$ and Pgp-1$^-$ subsets grow in response to optimal concentrations of recombinant IL-2 or IL-4 (Table 4). These preliminary data do not reveal any dramatic differences in lymphokine growth requirements between Pgp-1$^-$ and Pgp-1$^+$ T cells. More detailed studies involving dose-response analysis and ultimately lymphokine receptor binding assays will be required to determine whether quantitative differences do, however, exist in the responsiveness of these subsets to interleukins.

**Table 4.** Anti-CD3 induced proliferation of Pgp-1$^+$ and Pgp-1$^-$ subsets of CD8$^+$ T cells

| Subset | Anti-CD3 3 μg/ml | $^3$H-Thymidine incorporation (cpm ± SD) | | |
|---|---|---|---|---|
| | | Control | + IL-2 | + IL-4 |
| Pgp-1$^+$CD8$^+$ | − | 285 ± 159 | 2.451 ± 2628 | 183 ± 23 |
| | + | 365 ± 106 | 81.621 ± 13443 | 57.030 ± 9451 |
| Pgp-1$^-$CD8$^+$ | − | 303 ± 101 | 344 ± 127 | 281 ± 7982 |
| | + | 219 ± 33 | 140.175 ± 6.478 | 97.536 ± 7982 |

CD4-depleted lymph node cells from C57BL/6 mice were double stained with anti-Pgp-1 and anti-CD8 mAbs (see Fig. 1) and sterilely sorted into Pgp-1$^+$CD8$^+$ and Pgp-1$^-$CD8$^+$ subsets. Sorted cells (500 per microwell) were plated into control microwells or microwells that had been pretreated with anti-CD3 mAb 145-2C11 (LEO et al. 1987) at an optimal final concentration of 3 μg IgG/ml. Cultures were supplemented with IL-2 (60 ng/ml) or IL-4 (10 ng/ml) where indicated. $^3$H-Thymidine (1 μCi/well) was added overnight on day 5–6

## 3.7 Nonspecific Cytolysis

Activated CD8$^+$ T cells are capable of nonspecifically lysing tumor target cells in the presence of lectins or anti-TCR antibodies. When Pgp-1$^+$ and Pgp-1$^-$ subsets of CD8$^+$ cells were compared in this latter assay (following activation by anti-CD3 mAbs plus lymphokines), no significant differences were observed (Fig. 3). In particular, both subsets acquired equivalent levels of nonspecific cytolytic function when grown in the presence of IL-2 or IL-4. In all cases, cytolysis was TCR-dependent since it required the presence of anti-CD3 mAbs during the assay. It thus appears that the increased antigen-specific cytolytic function of recently activated Pgp-1$^+$ T cells (see Sect. 3.2) reflects an enrichment of specifically activated cells in the Pgp-1$^+$ fraction rather than an intrinsically enhanced cytolytic capacity. Such a conclusion is consistent with many studies of antigen-specific T-cell clones, where there is no consistent correlation between cytolytic capacity (i.e., lysis at a given effector to target ratio) and TCR affinity (as measured indirectly by anti-CD8 mAb inhibition). In any case, utilization of anti-CD3 mAb (bound to Fc receptors on P-815 target cells) to trigger nonspecific cytolysis in our system may circumvent any potential differences in cytolytic capacity, even if they were to exist.

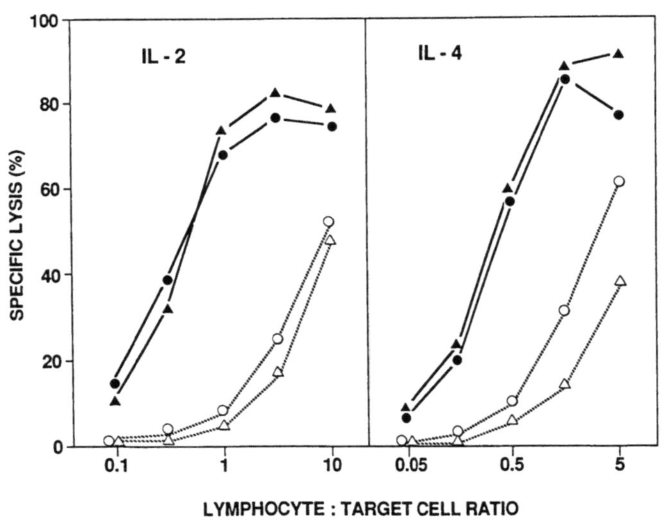


**Fig. 3.** Cytolytic activity of Pgp-1$^+$ and Pgp-1$^-$ subsets of CD8$^+$ T lymphocytes. CD4-depleted nylon wool purified lymph node cells from C57BL/6 mice were stained and sorted as in Table 4. Sorted cells (500 per well) were cultured on anti-CD3 mAb coated plates in the presence of either IL-2 60 ng/ml (*left panel*) or IL-4 10 ng/ml (*right panel*). On day 7, CD8$^+$ Pgp-1$^+$ (*circles*) and CD8$^+$ Pgp-1$^-$ (*triangles*) cells were assayed for cytolytic activity against $^{51}$Cr-labeled P-815 target cells in the presence (*filled symbols*) or absence (*open symbols*) of anti-CD3 mAb (Leo et al. 1987). Data are presented as percentage specific lysis at various lymphocyte to target cell ratios

# 4 Stability of Pgp-1 Phenotype

An important question arising from these studies in whether the Pgp-1 antigen is a stable phenotypic marker. To address this issue, sorted Pgp-1$^+$ and Pgp-1$^-$ T cells were stimulated in vitro with mitogens or alloantigens at limiting dilution and reanalyzed for Pgp-1 expression (BUDD et al. 1987b). It was found that both populations were virtually 100% Pgp-1$^+$ at 7 days and that this phenotype was stable for as long as the cultures could be viably maintained without restimulation (22 days). A more detailed kinetic analysis of acquisition of Pgp-1 was performed on CRT (95% Pgp-1$^-$ initially). Here, weak Pgp-1 expression by the majority of cells was seen 24 h after stimulation, and maximal expression was seen by 3 days. It thus appears that stable expression of Pgp-1 (at least in vitro) occurs concomitantly with antigenic (or mitogenic) stimulation.

The stability of Pgp-1 expression in vivo is a more difficult question to assess. However, several indirect arguments favor the hypothesis that Pgp-1 is also acquired in vivo following an encounter with antigen. As mentioned previously (Table 1), the majority (> 95%) of thymocytes with a mature (CD4$^+$ or CD8$^+$) phenotype are Pgp-1$^-$, whereas peripheral T cells contain a significant proportion (20%–40%)of Pgp-1$^+$ cells. This proportion of Pgp-1$^+$ peripheral T cells increases with age and undergoes a striking increase following adult thymectomy (BUDD et al. 1987b). Furthermore, T cells in congenitally athymic (nude) mice are almost exclusively of the Pgp-1$^+$ phenotype. These data thus demonstrate that the presence of peripheral Pgp-1$^-$ T cells is thymus dependent, consistent with the hypothesis that thymus emigrants are responsible for renewal of peripheral lymphoid tissues. However, they do not directly address the issue of whether Pgp-1$^-$ cells become Pgp-1$^+$ following antigenic stimulation.

The latter notion is supported for CD8$^+$ T cells by more careful analysis of the frequency and "affinity" of antigen-specific cytolytic T-lymphocyte precursors (CTLp) in alloimmunized mice (BUDD et al. 1987a, b). Thus, CTLp bearing putative high-affinity TCR (and consequently resistant to inhibition by anti-CD8

**Table 5.** Frequency of "high-affinity" (anti-CD8-resistant) CTLp in Pgp-1 subsets of spleen cells from normal or alloimmune C57BL/6 mice

| Immunization | Subset | CTLp frequency (reciprocal) | |
|---|---|---|---|
| | | Total | Anti-CD8 resistant |
| None | Pgp-1$^-$ | 41 | 242 |
| | Pgp-1$^+$ | 49 | 221 |
| Allo MHC | Pgp-1$^-$ | 49 | 1649 |
| | Pgp-1$^+$ | 15 | 22 |

Anti-H-2$^d$ CTLp frequencies were measured by limiting dilution in the presence or absence of anti-CD8 mAbs. For further details see BUDD et al. (1987b)

mAbs) were enriched (fourfold) in the Pgp-1$^+$ subset of alloimmune mice and depleted (sevenfold) in the Pgp-1$^-$ subset, despite the fact that the overall CTLp frequency in the latter subset remain unchanged (Table 5). In contrast, the proportion of allospecific CTLp bearing putative high-affinity TCR was identical in the Pgp-1$^+$ and Pgp-1$^-$ subsets of control (unimmunized) mice. Such a result is consistent with selection (by antigen) of CTLp bearing high-affinity TCR that subsequently acquire Pgp-1 during the course of their differentiation to memory cells in vivo.

## 5 Function of the Pgp-1 Molecule

Another issue arising from these studies is whether the Pgp-1 molecule itself mediates a specific function. Since memory T cells in man express enhanced levels of several molecules involved in activation or adhesion (such as CD2, LFA-1 and LFA-3; see SANDERS et al. 1988), we tested the effect of anti-Pgp-1 mAbs on T-cell-mediated cytolysis. As shown in Fig. 4, no inhibition of cytolysis by anti-Pgp-1 mAbs was observed, even under conditions where cell interaction was made limiting by addition of cytolysis-inhibiting doses of mAbs directed against CD8

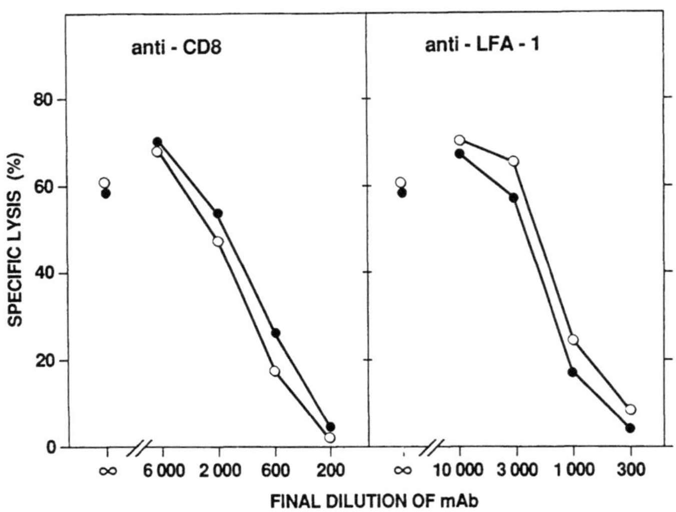


**Fig. 4.** Lack of inhibition of T-cell-mediated cytolysis by anti-Pgp-1 mAb. C57BL/6 anti-H-2K$^d$ cytolytic clone 860/7 (J. MARYANSKI and H.R. MACDONALD, unpublished data) was assayed for cytotoxicity against $^{51}$Cr-labeled P-815 (H-2$^d$) target cells at a 3:1 effector to target ratio. mAbs directed against CD8 (53-6.7; LEDBETTER and HERZENBERG 1979) or LFA-1 (FD 18.5; SARMIENTO et al. 1982) were added at the indicated dilutions in the presence (*filled symbols*) or absence (*open symbols*) of a saturating concentration of anti-Pgp-1 mAb IM 7.8.1 (1:3 culture supernatant). Specific lysis was assessed after 3 h. Similar data were obtained with four other CTL clones

or LFA-1. In other experiments, we have also failed to activate T cells with anti-Pgp-1 mAbs (unpublished data). Thus the Pgp-1 epitope recognized by mAb IM 7.8.1 may not be involved in activation or adhesion.

## 6 Concluding Remarks

The data summarized in this communication led to a simplified model for the cellular differentiation pathway leading to the formation of memory T lymphocytes. Thus mature "virgin" T cells produced in the thymus (Pgp-$1^-$) seed the peripheral lymphoid tissues. Following an encounter with antigen, these T cells are selected according to the affinity of their antigen receptors. Those with sufficiently high affinity TCR to be triggered acquire Pgp-1 expression as they differentiate into effector and (ultimately) memory T cells. Once acquired, Pgp-1 expression would be stable for the lifetime of the cell.

Such a model has several interesting implications regarding the T-cell repertoire. First, the presence of a significant proportion of Pgp-$1^+$ T lymphocytes in normal adult mice would be predicted to be a consequence of natural immunization to environmental antigens. Furthermore, the fact that allospecific CTLp in unprimed mice are equally frequent (and express equivalently avid TCR) in both Pgp-$1^-$ and Pgp-$1^+$ subsets is a strong argument in favor of the idea that environmentally primed T cells have a broad cross-reactivity to MHC determinants.

Finally, despite current lack of knowledge of the function of the Pgp-1 glycoprotein, it is clear that Pgp-1 represents a useful marker for the identification and separation of T lymphocytes with the expected properties of memory cells.

*Acknowledgements.* We wish to thank C. Horvath, C. Bron, T. Pedrazzini, and R.C. Howe who collaborated in various aspects of this work as well as A.-F. Brunet for preparing the manuscript. Recombinant human IL-2 and murine IL-4 were generously provided by Biogen S.A. (Geneva, Switzerland) and Immunex Corporation (Seattle, Washington, USA) respectively.

## References

Andersson B (1970) Studies of the regulation of avidity at the level of the single antibody-forming cell. The effect of antigen dose and time after immunization. J Exp Med 132: 77

Berke G, Sullivan KA, Amos DB (1972) Rejection of ascites tumor allograft. I. Isolation, characterization and in vitro reactivity of peritoneal effector cells from Balb/c mice immune to EL-4 leukosis. J Exp Med 135: 1334

Budd RC, Cerottini J-C, MacDonald HR (1987a) Phenotypic identification of memory cytolytic T lymphocytes in a subset of Lyt-$2^+$ cells. J Immunol 138: 1009

Budd RC, Cerottini J-C, Horvath C, Bron C, Pedrazzini T, Howe RC, MacDonald HR (1987b) Distinction of virgin and memory T lymphocytes. Stable acquisition of the Pgp-1 glycoprotein concomitant with antigenic stimulation. J Immunol 138: 3120
Budd RC, Cerottini J-C, MacDonald HR (1987c) Selectively increased production of interferon-γ by subsets of Lyt-$2^+$ and L3T$4^+$ T cells identified by expression of Pgp-1. J Immunol 138: 3583–86
Butterfield K, Fathman CG, Budd RC (1989) A subset of memory CD$4^+$ helper T lymphocytes identified by expression of Pgp-1. J Exp Med 169: 1461
Celada F (1971) The cellular basis of the immunologic memory. Prog Allergy 15: 223
Cerottini J-C, Brunner KT (1974) Cell-mediated cytotoxicity, allograft rejection and tumor immunity. Adv Immunol 18: 67
Cerottini J-C, MacDonald HR (1989) The cellular basis of T cell memory. Annu Rev Immunol 7: 77
Colombatti A, Hughes EN, Taylor BA, August JT (1982) Gene for a major cell surface glycoprotein of mouse macrophages and other phagocytic cells is on chromosome 2. Proc Natl Acad Sci USA 79: 1926
Davie JM, Paul WE (1972) Receptors on immunocompetent cells. V. Cellular correlations of the "maturation" of the immune response. J Exp Med 135: 660
Eisen HN, Siskind GW (1964) Variations in affinities of antibodies during the immune response. Biochemistry 3: 996
Golstein P, Goridis C, Schmitt-Verhulst A-M, Hayot B, Pierres A, van Agthoven A, Kaufmann Y, Eshhar Z, Pierres M (1982) Lymphoid cell surface interaction structures detected using cytolysis-inhibiting monoclonal antibodies. Immunol Rev 68: 5
Hughes EN, Mengod G, August JT (1981) Murine cell surface glycoproteins. Characterization of a major component of 80000 daltons as a polymorphic differentiation antigen of mesenchymal cells. J Biol Chem 256: 7023
Hughes EN, Colombatti A, August JT (1983) Murine cell surface glycoproteins. Purification of the polymorphic Pgp-1 antigen and analysis of its expression on macrophages and other myeloid cells. J Biol Chem 258: 1014
Ledbetter JA, Herzenberg LA (1979) Xenogeneic monoclonal antibodies to mouse lymphoid differentiation antigens. Immunol Rev 47: 63
Leo O, Foo M, Sachs DH, Samelson LE, Bluestone JA (1987) Identification of a monoclonal antibody specific for murine T3. Proc Natl Acad Sci USA 84: 1374
Lesley J, Hyman R, Schulte R (1985a) Evidence that the Pgp-1 glycoprotein is expressed on thymus-homing progenitor cells of the thymus. Cell Immunol 91: 397
Lesley J, Trotter J, Hyman R (1985b) The Pgp-1 antigen is expressed on early fetal thymocytes. Immunogenetics 22: 149
Lesley J, Schulte R, Trotter J, Hyman R (1988) Qualitative and quantitative heterogeneity in Pgp-1 expression among murine thymocytes. Cell Immunol 112: 40
Lynch F, Ceredig R (1988) Ly-24 (Pgp-1) expression by thymocytes and peripheral T cells. Immunol Today 9: 7
Lynch F, Chaudhri G, Allan JE, Doherty PC, Ceredig R (1987) Expression of Pgp-1 (or Ly24) by subpopulations of mouse thymocytes and activated peripheral T lymphocytes. Eur J Immunol 17: 137
MacDonald HR, Cerottini J-C, Ryser J-E, Maryanski JL, Taswell C, Widmer MB, Brunner KT (1980) Quantitation and cloning of cytolytic T lymphocytes and their precursors. Immunol Rev 51: 93
MacDonald HR, Glasebrook AL, Bron C, Kelso A, Cerottini J-C (1982) Clonal heterogeneity in the functional requirement for Lyt-2/3 molecules on cytolytic T lymphocytes (CTL): possible implications for the affinity of CTL antigen receptors. Immunol Rev 68: 89
Marrack P, Endres R, Shimonkevitz R, Zlotnik A, Dialynas D, Fitch FW, Kappler J (1983) The major histocompatibility complex-restricted antigen receptor on T cells. II. Role of the L3T4 product. J Exp Med 158: 1077
Miethke T, Schmidberger R, Heeg K, Gillis S, Wagner H (1988) Interleukin 4 (BSF-1) induces growth in resting murine CD8 T cells triggered via cross-linking of T3 cell surface structures. Eur J Immunol 18: 767
Mosmann TR, Coffman RL (1987) Two types of mouse helper T-cell clone. Immunol Today 8: 223
Sanders ME, Makgoba MW, Sharrow SO, Stephany D, Springer TA, Young HA, Shaw S (1988) Human memory T lymphocytes express increased levels of three cell adhesion molecules (LFA-3, CD2, and LFA-1) and three other molecules (UCHLI, CDw29, and Pgp-1) and have enhanced IFN-γ production. J Immunol 140: 1401
Sarmiento M, Dialynas DP, Lancki DW, Wall KA, Lorber MI, Loken MR, Fitch FW (1982) Cloned

T lymphocytes and monoclonal antibodies as probes for cell surface molecules active in T cell-mediated cytolysis. Immunol Rev 68: 135

Schmidberger R, Miethke T, Heeg K, Wagner H (1988) Primary activation of murine CD8 T cells via cross-linking of T3 cell surface structures: two signals regulate induction of IL-2 responsiveness. Eur J Immunol 18: 277

Shimonkevitz R, Luescher B, Cerottini J-C, MacDonald HR (1985) Clonal analysis of cytolytic T lymphocyte-mediated lysis of target cells with inducible antigen expression: correlation between antigen density and requirement for Lyt-2/3 function. J Immunol 135: 892

Swain SL (1983) T cell subsets and the recognition of MHC class. Immunol Rev 74: 129

Taniguchi T (1988) Regulation of cytokine gene expression. Annu Rev Immunol 6: 439

Trowbridge IS, Lesley J, Schulte R, Hyman R, Trotter J (1982) Biochemical characterization and cellular distribution of a polymorphic, murine cell-surface glycoprotein expressed on lymphoid cells. Immunogenetics 15: 299

Trowbridge IS, Lesley J, Trotter J, Hyman R (1985) Thymocyte subpopulation enriched for progenitors with an unrearranged T-cell receptor $\beta$-chain gene. Nature 315: 666

# Human T-Cell Memory

P. C. L. BEVERLEY



## 1 Introduction

The specificity and memory of immune responses sets them apart from all other physiological responses except those of the nervous system. These properties have long been recognised by immunologists, and while specificity is well accounted for by clonally distributed B- and T-cell receptors, the nature of immunological memory still poses many problems. While it has often been assumed that memory cells are long-lived and not dependent on continuous or repeated antigenic stimulation, this view has been challenged by recent data which suggest that persistence of memory is dependent on continued antigen drive (GRAY and SKARVALL 1988).

For B cells, development of an antibody response and memory is associated with isotype switching and changes in affinity. The molecular genetic mechanisms

Imperial Cancer Research Fund Human Tumour Immunology Group, University College and Middlesex School of Medicine, The Courtauld Institute of Biochemistry, 91 Riding House Street, London WIP 8BT, UK

Current Topics in Microbiology and Immunology, Vol. 159

underlying these events in B cells have been well studied (CUMANO et al. 1986; CEBRA et al. 1984). In contrast, neither changes in isotype or affinity have been described for T-cell responses during the development of effector or memory cells. It is thus of particular interest to determine in what way memory cells differ from unprimed cells and how this affects the nature of primary and memory T-cell responses.

In humans, ethical constraints inhibit experimental investigation of the development of memory. Counterbalancing this difficulty for immunologists, however, is the advantage of having a very large number of phenotypic markers available for human lymphocytes. It is these markers which have allowed the definition of unprimed and memory T-cell populations in humans. The results of studies in man now also receive support from experiments in rodents, although the phenotypic analysis is less complete in the mouse and rat.

## 2 Definition of T-Cell Memory

In this review the operational definition of T memory cells which we use is "those cells which respond in vitro to antigens to which the individual has previously been exposed". Such a definition raises several questions. In particular, what are cells which do not respond to such antigens? Are they unprimed T cells or a subset of cells which fail to respond under the particular in vitro conditions used? This question might be more readily answered if primary T-cell responses could be reliably obtained in man. However, although primary humoral responses have been described (MORIMOTO et al. 1986), in most cases there is little information as to the nature of the T cells involved, and it is difficult in adult humans to exclude the possibility that the responses are in reality mediated by cells primed by cross-reacting antigens. We will therefore have little to say about primary T-cell responses to specific antigens, but both rodent data and evidence from phenotypic changes in vitro strongly suggest a maturation sequence leading from cells unable to respond to recall antigens to cells with a phenotype characteristic of those responding to recall antigens (memory cells;

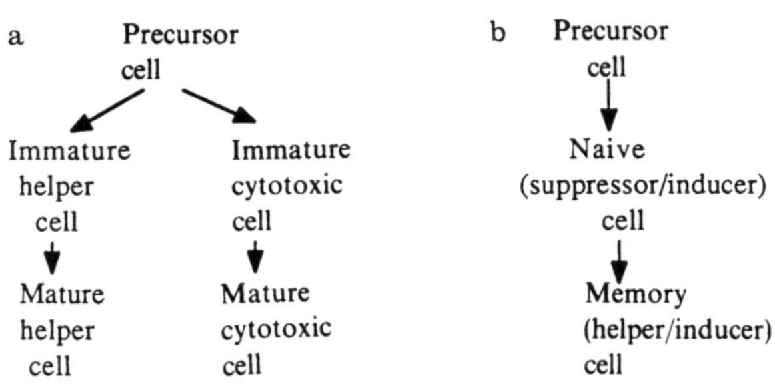


**Fig. 1. a** Lineage relationship of T-cell subsets. **b** Maturational relationship of T-cell subsets

Fig. 1b). In our studies we have examined responses to the recall antigens tetanus toxoid, influenza virus, purified protein derivative (PPD) and Epstein-Barr virus (EBV). While in most cases we have no direct evidence that our donors have been exposed to these antigens, it is very likely that they have.

## 3 Human T-Cell Heterogeneity

Monoclonal antibodies (mAbs) have provided numerous reagents to investigate the function of human T cells. Although other methods allowed some separation of human T-cell subsets (EVANS et al. 1977; MORETTA et al. 1977), the wider availability of mAbs has the advantage that results obtained from different laboratories are more comparable. However, even mAbs belonging to the same cluster of differentiation (CD) may not always give exactly the same results, particularly when used to stimulate or block function (MEUER et al. 1984). Because of their differing functional effects, even when used in cell separation procedures, individual mAbs may have distinct effects on the separated cells. Such effects may in part account for differences between laboratories.

Many mAbs have been used to study human T-cell heterogeneity (Table 1). The initial separation into the largely non-overlapping CD4 and CD8 subsets with distinct properties and genetic restriction has been confirmed and extended in many laboratories (REINHERZ and SCHLOSSMAN 1980). While co-expression of the CD4 and CD8 antigens on peripheral T cells has been described (BLUE et al. 1985), the importance of this remains uncertain, and there is little evidence of interconversion between CD4 and CD8 cells. Thus, these two subpopulations may be considered to be stable sublineages of T cells, presumably originating from a thymic double positive precursor (Fig. 1a).

Within the CD4 and CD8 subsets, the significance of the further heterogeneity in antigen expression detected by the mAbs listed in Table 1 is less clear; there are

**Table 1.** Antigenic heterogeneity of CD4

| Antibody | Marker for | Reference |
|---|---|---|
| CD45RA (eg., 2H4) | Suppressor/inducer or naive cells | Morimoto et al. 1985a |
| CD45RO (eg., UCHL1) | Helper/inducer or memory cells | Smith et al. 1986 |
| CD29 | Subset of helper/inducer or memory cells | Morimoto et al. 1985b |
| 5.9 | Subset of helper/inducer or memory cells | Corte et al. 1982 |
| Ta1 | Subset of helper/inducer or memory cells | Hafler et al. 1986 |
| D44 | Subset of helper/inducer of memory cells | Calvo et al. 1986 |
| CD28 (eg., 9.3) | Helpers, $CTL_p$ and CTL | Lum et al. 1982 |
| Leu 8 | Most CD45R, subset of memory cells | Gatenby et al. 1982 |
| TQ1 | Similar to Leu 8 | Reinherz et al. 1982 |
| LFA-3 (CD56) | Memory cells | Sanders et al. 1988 |
| I-CAM-1 (CD54) | Memory cells | Buckle and Hogg 1989 |

Most of these antigens are not T-cell specific

several possibilities. Phenotypic differences might indicate further distinct sublineages or identify stages of maturation. They might be related to cell cycle or be expressed as a consequence of the local environment in blood or lymphoid tissue. For many antigens the picture remains unclear, but we shall argue that expression of different isoforms of CD45 is closely linked to maturation of T cells in both the CD4 and CD8 sublineages.

## 4 CD45

The CD45 (leucocyte common) antigen is a complex of high molecular weight polypeptides expressed on all leucocytes. There is a single CD45 gene, but several isoforms can be produced by alternative splicing of exons near the N-terminus of the molecule (Fig. 2). In humans four different types of antibody to CD45 have been identified. Conventional CD45 mAbs bind to all isoforms while one mAb against exon B immunoprecipitates three polypeptides. CD45RA mAbs against exon A react with 220 kDa and 205 kDa polypeptides while the CD45RO mAb UCHL1 reacts only with a 180 kDa polypeptide (STREULI et al. 1987). Among T cells, CD45RA and CD45RO mAbs identify largely non-overlapping subpopulations (MORIMOTO et al. 1985a; SMITH et al. 1986).

MAbs to CD45 have been shown to interfere with or potentiate many lymphocyte functions (reviewed in TIGHE et al. 1987). These data remained difficult to interpret until the recent discovery that the cytoplasmic domain of CD45 functions as a tyrosine phosphatase (CHARBONNEAU et al. 1988). Cross-linking experiments have shown that approximation of CD45 to other molecules, such as CD3, on the cell surface can strongly inhibit signal transduction (LEDBETTER et al. 1988). The implication of these data is that CD45 is an important cell surface signalling molecule, though the function of the different isoforms remains to be determined.

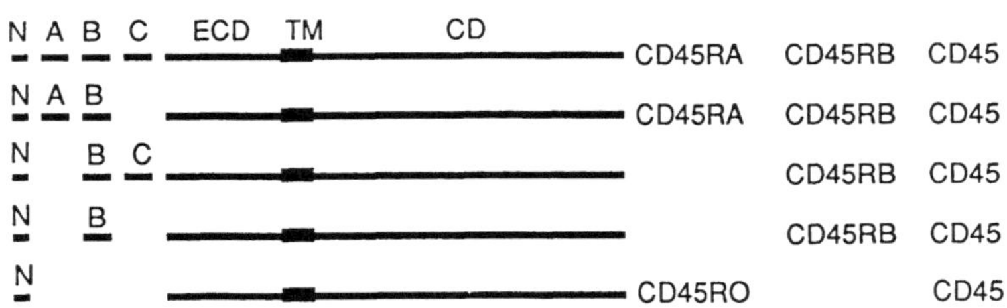


**Fig. 2.** Alternative splicing of CD45. *A B* and *C* are exons toward the N-terminus of the extracellular domain (*ECD*) of CD45 which can be alternatively spliced to give the different isoforms shown. *N* is the short N-terminal sequence present in all isoforms. The cytoplasmic domain (*CD*) has homology to a recently described tyrosine phosphatase. *TM*, transmembrane sequence

## 5 Function of CD45RA and CD45RO T Cells

Several laboratories have examined the functions of CD45RA and CD45RO T-cell subsets (e.g. MORIMOTO et al. 1985a; SMITH et al. 1986; TEDDER et al. 1985). Many of these data relate to CD4, and the results can be summarised as follows: Both subsets respond equally in mixed lymphocyte cultures (MLC) and proliferate well in response to non-specific mitogens such as phytohaemagglutinin (PHA), but only the CD45RO population responds to soluble antigens (MORIMOTO et al. 1985a; SMITH et al. 1986). The CD45RA population responds better in the auto-mixed lymphocyte reaction (MLR) than does the CD45RO population. Only the CD45RO population can provide help for pokeweed mitogen (PWM)-driven immunoglobulin synthesis or a specific antibody response (MORIMOTO et al. 1986; BEVERLEY et al. 1986). In the PWM model, CD45RA-expressing cells have been shown to induce suppression (MORIMOTO et al. 1985a).

These data can be interpreted either as indicating two sublineages within the CD4 subset or as separating unprimed (CD45RA) from memory (CD45RO) cells. If the former is correct, the lack of antigen-specific reactivity to recall antigens is puzzling. Our own attempts by limiting dilution analysis, with or without addition of cytokines and removal of CD8-expressing ($CD8^+$) cells, failed to indicate antigen-specific responses of $CD45RA^+$ cells (MERKENSCHLAGER et al. 1988). These experiments did show a large difference in precursor frequency for responses to soluble recall antigens, but no difference in frequency of alloreactive precursors. We concluded that these experiments indicate that $CD45RA^+$ $CD4^+$ cells represent an unprimed population and that memory $CD4^+$ T cells express CD45RO (Fig. 1b). A clear prediction of this view is that $CD45RA^+$ cells should express CD45RO following activation. This has been shown to occur following PHA allostimulation (AKBAR et al. 1988; SERRA et al. 1988). The expression of CD45RA declines at the same time.

There is much less data available with regard to the function of CD8 subsets detected by CD45RA and RO mAbs. However, we have recently shown that both subsets can generate allospecific cytotoxic cells (CTLs) while only $UCHL1^+$ (CD45RO) cells generate EBV-specific restricted CTLs (MERKENSCHLAGER and BEVERLEY 1989). Limiting dilution analysis of CTL precursor (CTLp) frequency gave straight lines in Poisson analysis, suggesting that no other cell type was required for generation of CTL from CTLp. The frequency of CTLp among $CD45RO^+$ T cells varied between 1:16000 and 1:49000 while in the CD45RA population it was > 1:100000. We further showed that in bulk cultures $CD8^+$ $UCHL1^+$ cells alone were able to generate CTLs when stimulated with autologous EBV lymphoblastoid cell lines (EBV-LCL). This is in line with earlier data suggesting that $CD8^+$ cells alone are capable of inducing regression of autologous EBV-infected B cells (CRAWFORD et al. 1983). It appears therefore that in both CD4 and CD8 populations, maturation from an unprimed CD45RA to a memory CD45RO population occurs. Such a transition is strongly supported by recent experiments in the rat in which T cells responding in primary and secondary humoral responses can be distinguished by the expression of different CD45 isoforms (POWRIE and MASON 1988).

## 6 Properties of Naive and Memory T Cells

We have chosen to use mAbs to CD45 isoforms to separate T cells with high expression of CD45RA or CD45RO because this allows isolation of either population by negative selection, so that the cells do not carry over bound mAb into the in vitro cultures. However, other mAbs have been used to achieve separation of functionally similar subpopulations (MORIMOTO et al. 1985b; SANDERS et al. 1988; BUCKLE and HOGG 1989). Thus, it has become clear that naive and memory T cells not only differ in expression of CD45 isoforms but also show major quantitative differences in the expression of several other surface antigens (Table 2). We have confirmed these results by double staining unseparated T cell or by restaining negatively selected CD45RA and RO expressing cells. Figure 3 shows fluorescence-activated cell sorter (FACS) profiles of the two populations stained with mAbs against several of the mAbs of Table 2.

It is notable that most of the antigens showing higher expression on memory cells have been shown to be important in cell-cell interactions (adhesion molecules; SPRINGER et al. 1987; SHAW et al. 1986). CD2 is also capable of delivering an activation signal to T cells (MEUER et al. 1984). It is therefore hardly surprising that functional differences between the CD45RA and RO populations have been noted in proliferative responses to CD2 and CD3 mAbs. Three groups of workers have shown strong responses by CD45RO$^+$ cells and weak responses by CD45RA$^+$ cells to CD2 mAbs (SANDERS et al. 1988; HUET et al. 1988; WALLACE and BEVERLEY, unpublished data). A contrary result, not so far readily explicable, has however been obtained by MORIMOTO (1988). Two groups of workers show stronger responses to CD3 mAbs by CD45RO than CD45RA

**Table 2.** Phenotype of virgin and memory T cells

| Phenotype | Virgin cells (Suppressor/ inducers) | Memory cells (helper/ inducers) |
|---|---|---|
| CD45R | ++ | — |
| UCHL1 | — | ++ |
| CDw29 | — | ++ |
| Pgp-1 | + | ++ |
| CD18/CD11a | + | ++ |
| CD2 | + | ++ |
| LFA-3 | + | ++ |

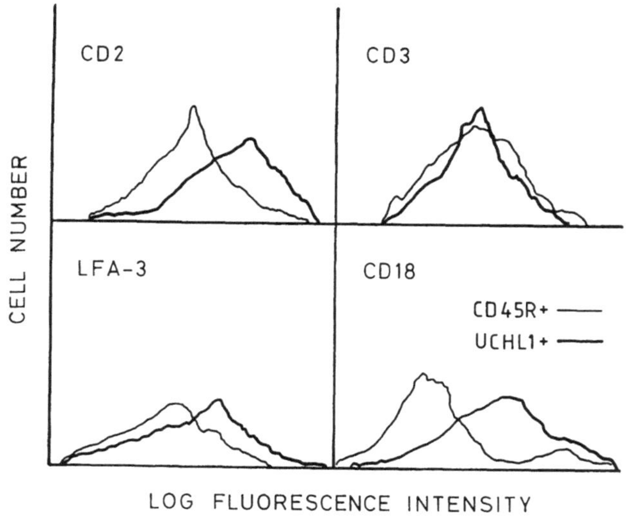


**Fig. 3.** Fluorescence histograms of CD45R$^+$ and UCHL1$^+$ cells separated by negative selection from sheep red cell rosette positive cells using magnetic beads. The small population of CD45R$^+$ cells brightly stained with CD18 are NK cells

populations (SANDERS et al. 1988; BYRNE et al. 1988), while others find no consistent differences (MORIMOTO 1988; WALLACE and BEVERLEY, unpublished data). Again the differences are not readily explicable but may relate to differences in mAbs used for activation, separation procedures or culture conditions. Perhaps more persuasive than these differences in non-specific responses is the observation that memory cells make a more rapid response in alloresponses than do naive cells (LECHLER, personal communication). Thus, high expression of adhesion molecules does influence the function of naive and virign cells.

These and other molecules such as CD29 and CD44 may play a role in determining the migration patterns of CD45RA and CD45RO expressing T cells. CD29 is one of the $\beta$-chains of the integrin family of molecules which plays a role in platelet adhesion (Leucocyte Typing Workshop 1989). Studies of T-cell endothelial interactions confirm that CD45RO$^+$ cells adhere more readily to endothelia than do CD45RA$^+$ cells (CAVENDER et al. 1988), and other studies indicate that inflammatory lesions generally contain more UCHL1$^+$ than CD45RA$^+$ cells (PIZALIS et al. 1987). It may be, therefore, that memory cells enter tissues more readily, although activation of CD45RA$^+$ cells in inflammatory sites may contribute to the preponderance of CD45RO$^+$ cells.

While rodent data on the phenotypes of naive and memory cells is less extensive than in man, increased expression of Pgp-1, the murine homologue of CD44, has been shown to characterise memory T cells in at least some strains of mice (BUDD et al. 1987).

# 7 Unresolved Problems

## 7.1 Alloresponses and Recall Responses

Although much of the published data on T-cell heterogeneity is interpretable as detection of maturation stages within the major CD4 and CD8 sublineages of T cells, some observations remain difficult to accommodate within such a framework. Our own limiting dilution analysis shows that both naive and memory T cells respond with equal frequency to alloantigens. Responses of memory cells to alloantigens presumably represent cross-reactions; this phenomenon has been demonstrated for many T-cell clones (ASHWELL et al. 1986). It is thus puzzling that responses to alloantigens and to soluble recall antigens can be isolated in the small $5.9^{+}$ subset (HAFLER et al. 1986). These results are reminiscent of earlier rat data which appeared to separate alloresponses and recall responses (ARTHUR and MASON 1986) but which can now be better attributed to differences in the tissue culture requirements of naive and memory T cells (POWRIE and MASON 1988). Whether $5.9^{-}$ cells have similarly distinct culture requirements or whether they are unable to produce sufficient interleukins for proliferation remains to be determined.

## 7.2 Subsets of Memory Cells

In the mouse, two distinct categories of $CD4^{+}$ T-cell clones have been described (MOSSMANN et al. 1986), differing in their lymphokine production. Predominantly $T_H1$ or $T_H2$ clones are obtained by different immunisation schedules. It is at present unclear whether these different helper cell types represent sublineages of CD4 or whether all T cells can pass through successive stages in vivo, expressing $T_H1$- or $T_H2$-like properties. $T_H1$ and $T_H2$ clones maintained in vitro would, according to the latter view, represent T cells "frozen" at different stages of maturation. In man too it is unclear whether phenotypic heterogeneity of CD45RO expressing cells detected with, for example, Leu8 or CD29 represents sublineages or further steps in maturation. Human T-cell clones are heterogeneous with respect to cytokine production (PALIARD et al. 1988), though two broad categories, differing in cytolytic activity and the spectrum of cytokines produced, have been described (ROTTEVEEL et al. 1988). Among freshly isolated T cells, considerable differences in cytokine production can also be detected following separation of various subsets (SALMON et al. 1988; HEDLUND et al. 1989).

## 7.3 Suppression and Suppressor Induction

The nature of suppression remains in doubt at present. In humans suppression of PWM and auto-MLC-induced immunoglobulin synthesis has been ascribed to

$CD8^+$ cells (MORIMOTO et al. 1985a; REINHERZ et al. 1980; LANDAY et al. 1983). Further separation into $CD28^+$ CTLs and CTLps and $CD11b^+$ suppressor cells has been documented (YAMADA et al. 1985), but suppression by $CD28^+$ cells has also been described (MORIMOTO et al. 1986). There is however little evidence of antigen-specific suppression in man, although low responders to several antigens may be converted to high responder status by removal of $CD8^+$ T cells. Our own limiting dilution experiments provide no evidence for the existence of suppressor cells in CD4 proliferative responses or generation of CTLs. At the present time it is difficult to put together the phenotypic data obtained mainly on non-specific suppressor cells with our own evidence for maturation of CD45RA to CD45RO among cytolytic cells. The possibility remains that suppression may be a function of $CD8^+$ cells expressed at a particular stage of maturation rather than of a distinct subset of cells, and this may also be the case for CD8-mediated amplification (HIROHATA et al. 1988).

Similar difficulties exist with respect to suppressor induction. $CD45RA^+$ cells have been shown in the PWM model to be necessary for the induction of CD8 suppressor activity (MORIMOTO et al. 1985a). One report documents a similar effect in an antigen-specific in vitro antibody response (MORIMOTO et al. 1986). However $CD45RA^+$ cells are not a stable subpopulation and become $CD45RO^+$ on stimulation, but there is so far little evidence that memory suppressor inducers exist (but see DAMLE et al. 1987). Thus, it seem likely either that suppressor induction is an in vitro artefact of the mitogen-driven pokeweed model or that suppressor induction is a transiently expressed function. There is some evidence that CD45RA and CD45RO expressing cells differ in cytokine production (SANDERS et al. 1988), lending some support to the latter view.

Both induction of suppression (HIRAYAMA et al. 1987) and the auto-MLC response have been linked to response to DQ (NIEDA et al. 1988) while the bulk of memory CD4 responses to most soluble antigens are DR restricted. This raises the question of whether there might be a large number of $CD45RA^+$ cells which are capable of responding to self-DQ and inducing suppression but which fail to mature to memory $CD45RO^+$ cells. This possibility remains to be examined.

## 8 Conclusion

Phenotypic analysis combined with in vitro assays has allowed the definition of two broad categories of cells among both the CD4 and CD8 sublineages of T cells. Naive (CD45RA) T cells express low levels of molecules known to be important in cell–cell interaction. This is likely to impose strict requirements for the initial activation of these cells. A second (CD45RO) population contains memory proliferative, helper and cytolytic precursor cells able to respond rapidly to recall antigens. It remains unclear whether the naive population contains precursors pre-committed to becoming distinct effector cell types (e.g., $T_H1$ and

$T_H2$ or cytotoxic and suppressor cells) or whether the mode of antigen presentation determines the outcome of a primary T-cell response. At the memory level, considerable phenotypic and functional heterogeneity is demonstrable, but at present it is uncertain if this represents further antigen-driven stages of maturation within this cell pool or the development of different sublineages of $CD4^+$ or $CD8^+$ T cells.

## References

Akbar AN, Terry LA, Timms A, Beverley PCL, Janossy G (1988) Loss of CD45R and gain of UCHL1 reactivity is a feature of primed T cells. J Immunol 140: 2171–2179
Arthur RP, Mason D (1986) T cells that help B cell responses to soluble antigen are distinguishable from those producing interleukin 2 on mitogenic or allogenec stimulation. J Exp Med 163: 774–786
Ashwell JD, Chen C, Schwartz RH (1986) High frequency and non-random distribution of alloreactivity in T cell clones selected for recognition of foreign antigen in association with self class II molecules. J Immunol 136: 389–395
Beverley PCL, Terry L, Pickford A (1986) T cell subsets and function. In: Cinader B, Miller R (eds) Progress in immunology VI. Academic, Orlando, pp 941–948
Blue ML, Daley JF, Levine H, Schlossman SF (1985) Lectin activation induces T4, T8 co-expression on peripheral blood T cells. In: Reinherz EL et al. (eds) Leucocyte typing II. Springer, Berlin Heidelberg, New York, pp 89–100
Buckle A-M, Hogg N (1989) ICAM-1 expression on T cells. J Cell Biochem 13 A [Suppl] C109: 193
Budd RC, Cerottini J-C, MacDonald HR (1987) Phenotypic identification of memory cytolytic T lymphocytes in a subset of Lyt-2+ cells. J Immunol 138: 1009–1013
Byrne JA, Butler JL, Cooper M (1988) Differential activation requirements for virgin and memory T cells. J Immunol 141: 3249–3256
Calvo C-F, Bernard A, Huet S, Leroy E, Boumsell L, Senik A (1986) Regulation of immunoglobulin synthesis by human T cell subsets as defined by anti-D44 monoclonal antibody within the CD4+ and CD8+ subpopulations. J Immunol 136: 1144–1149
Cavender DE, Haskard DO, Maliakkai D, Ziff M (1987) Separation and characterisation of human T cell subsets with varying degrees of adhesiveness for endothelial cells (EC). Arthritis Rheum 30: 29–32
Cebra JJ, Komisar J-L, Schweitzer PA (1984) $C_h$ isotype "switching" during normal B-lymphocyte development. Annu Rev Immunol 2: 493–548
Charbonneau H, Tonks NK, Walsh KA, Fischer EH (1988). The leucocyte common antigen (CD45): a putative receptor-linked protein tyrosine phosphatase. Proc Natl Acad Sci USA 85: 7182–7186
Corte G, Mingari MC, Moretta A, Damiani G, Moretta L, Bargellesi A (1982) Human T cell subpopulations defined by a monoclonal antibody. I. A small subset is responsible for proliferation to allogeneic cells or to soluble antigens and for helper activity for B. J Immunol 128: 16–19
Crawford DH, Iliescu V, Edwards AJ, Beverley PCL (1983) Characterisation of Epstein Barr Virus-specific memory cells from the blood of seropositive individuals. J Cancer 47: 681–686
Cumano A, Dildrop R, Kocks C, Rajewsky K, Sablitzky F, Siekevitz M (1986) Mutation and selection of antibodies. In: Cinader B, Miller RG (eds) Progress in immunology VI. Academic, Orlando, pp 139–144
Damle NK, Childs AL, Doyle LV (1987) Immunoregulatory T lymphocytes in man. Soluble antigen-specific suppressor-inducer T lymphocytes are derived from the $CD4^+$ $CD45R\text{-}p80^+$ subpopulation. J Immunol 139: 1501–1508
Evans RL, Breard JM, Lazarus H, Schlossman SF, Chess L (1977) Detection, isolation and functional characterisation of two human T cell subclasses bearing unique differentiation antigens. J Exp Med 145: 221–228

Gatenby PA, Kansas GS, Xian CY, Evans RL, Engleman EG (1982) Dissection of immunoregulatory subpopulations of T lymphocytes within the helper and suppressor sublineages in man. J Immunol 129: 1997–2000
Gray D, Skarvall H (1988) B-cell memory is short-lived in the absence of antigen. Nature 336: 70–72
Hafler DA, Fox DA, Benjamin D, Weiner HL (1986) Antigen reactive memory cells are defined by Ta1 J Immunol 137: 414–418
Hedlund G, Dohlsten M, Sjogren HO, Carlsson R (1989) Maximal interferon-gamma production and early synthesis of interleukin-2 by CD4+Cdw29+CD45R-p80- human T lymphocytes. Immunology 66: 49–53
Hirayama K, Matsushita S, Kikuchi I, Iuchi M, Ohta N, Sasazuki T (1987) HLA-DQ is epistatic to HLA-DR in controlling the response to schistosomal antigens in humans. Nature 327: 426–429
Hirohata S, Jelinek DF, Lipsky PE (1988) T cell dependent activation of B cell proliferation and differentiation by immobilized monoclonal antibodies to CD3. J Immunol 140: 3720–3733
Huet S, Boumsell L, Dausset J, Degos L, Bernard A (1988) The required interaction between monocytes and peripheral blood T lymphocytes (T-PBL) upon activation via CD2 or CD3. Role of HLA class I molecules and the differential response of T-PBL subsets. Eur J Immunol 18: 1187–1194
Leucocyte typing IV. Proceedings of the 4th international workshop on leucocyte differentiation antigens (in preparation)
Landay A, Gartland GL, Clement LT (1983) Characterisation of a phenotypically distinct subpopulation of Leu 2+ cells that suppresses T cell proliferative responses. J Immunol 131: 2757–2763
Ledbetter JA, Tonks NK, Fischer EH, Clark EA (1988) CD45 regulates signal transduction and lymphocyte activation by specific association with receptor molecules on T or B cells. Proc Natl Acad Sci USA 85: 8628–8634
Lum LG, Orcutt-Thordarson N, Seineuret MC, Hansen JA (1982) In vitro regulation of immunoglobulin synthesis by T-cell subpopulations defined by a new human T-cell antigen (9.3). Cell Immunol 72: 122–129
Merkenschlager M, Beverley PCL (1989) Evidence for differential expression of CD45 isoforms by precursors for memory dependent and independent cytotoxic responses: Human CD8 memory CTLp selectively express CD45RO (UCHL1). International Immunol 1: 450– 459
Merkenschlager M, Terry L, Edwards R, Beverley PCL (1988) Limiting dilution analysis of proliferative responses in human lymphocyte populations defined by the monoclonal antibody UCHL1: implications for differential CD45 expression in T cells memory formation. Eur J Immunol 18: 1653–1659
Meuer SC, Hussey RE, Fabbi M, Fox D, Acuto O, Fitzgerald KA, Hodgdon JP, Protentis JP, Schlossman SF (1984) Alternative pathway of T-cell activation: a functional role for the 50 kd T11 sheep erythrocyte receptor protein. Cell 36: 897–908
Moretta L, Webb SR, Grossi CE, Lydyard PM, Cooper MD (1977) Functional analysis of two human T-cell subpopulations: help and suppression of B-cell responses by T cells bearing receptors for IgM or IgG. J Exp Med 146: 184–200
Morimoto C (1988) CD4+ CD45R + cells are preferentially activated through the CD2 pathway. Eur J Immunol 18: 473–1478
Morimoto C, Letvin NL, Distaso JA, Aldrich WR, Schlossman SF (1985a) The isolation and characterisation of the human suppressor inducer T cell subset. J Immunol 134: 1508–1515
Morimoto C, Letvin NL, Boyd AW, Hagan M, Brown HM, Kornacki MM, Schlossman SF (1985b) The isolation and characterisation of the human helper inducer T cell. subset. J Immunol 134: 3762–3769
Morimoto C, Letvin NL, Distaso JA, Brown HM, Schlossman SF (1986) The cellular basis for the induction of antigen-specific T8 suppressor cells. Eur J Immunol 16: 198–204
Mossmann TR, Cherwinski H, Bond MW, Giedlin MA, Coffman RL (1986) Two types of murine helper T cell clone. I. Definition according to profiles of lymphokine activities and secreted proteins. J Immunol 136: 2348–2357
Nieda M, Juji T, Imao S, Minami M (1988) A role of HLA-DQ molecules of stimulator-adherent cells in the regulation of human autologous mixed lymphocyte reaction. J Immunol 141: 2975–2979
Paliard X, De Waal Malefijt R, Yssel H, Blanchard D, Chretien I, Abrams J, De Vries J, Spits H (1988) Simultaneous production of IL-2, IL-4, and IFN-$\gamma$ by activated human $CD4^+$ and $CD8^+$ T cell clones. J Immunol 141: 849–855
Pizalis C, Kingsley G, Murphy J, Panayi G (1987) Abnormal distribution of the helper-inducer and

suppressor-inducer T-lymphocyte-subset in the rheumatoid joint. Clin Immunol Immunopathol 45: 252–258
Powrie F, Mason D (1988) The MRC OX-22⁻ CD4⁺ T cells that help B cells in secondary immune responses derive from naive precursors with the MRC OX-22⁺ CD4⁺ phenotype. J Exp Med 169: 653
Reinherz EL, Schlossman SF (1980) The differentiation and function of human T lymphocytes. Cell 19: 821–827
Reinherz EL, Morimoto C, Penta AC, Schlossman SF (1980) Regulation of B cell immunoglobulin secretion by functional subsets of T lymphocytes in man. Eur J Immunol 10: 570–572
Reinherz EL, Morimoto C, Fitzgerald KA, Hussey RE, Daley JF, Schlossmann SF (1982) Heterogeneity of human T4⁺ inducer T cells defined by a monoclonal antibody that delineates two functional subpopulations. J Immunol 126: 463–468
Rotteveel FTM, Kokkelink I, Van Lier RAW, Kuenen B, Meager A, Miedema F, Lucas CJ (1988) Clonal analysis of functionally distinct human CD4 + T cell subsets. J Exp Med 168: 1659–1674
Salmon M, Kitas GD, Hill Gaston JS, Bacon PA (1988) Interleukin-2 production and response by helper T-cell subsets in man. Immunology 65: 81–85
Sanders ME, Makgoba MW, Sharrow SO, Stephany D, Springer A, Young HA, Shaw S (1988a) Human memory T lymphocytes express increased levels of three cell adhesion molecules (LFA-3, CD-2, LFA-1) and three other molecules (UCHL1, CDw29 and Pgp-1) and have enhanced IFN-$\gamma$ production. J Immunol 140: 1401–1408
Sanders ME, Makgoba MW, Shaw S (1988b) Human naive and memory T cells: reinterpretation and further characterisation of helper-inducer and suppressor-inducer subsets. Immunol Today 9: 195–198
Serra HM, Krowka JF, Ledbetter JA, Pilarski LM (1988) Loss of CD45R (Lp220) represents a post-thymic T cell differentiation event. J Immunol 140: 1435–1442
Shaw S, Luce GEG, Quinones R, Gress RE, Springer TA, Sanders ME (1986) Two antigen-independent adhesion pathways used by human cytotoxic T cell clones. Nature 323: 262–265
Smith S, Brown MH, Rowe D, Callard RE, Beverley PCL (1986) Functional subsets of human helper-inducer cells defined by a new mAb, UCHL1. Immunology 58: 63–70
Springer TA, Dunstin ML, Kishimoto TK, Marlin SD (1987) The lymphocyte function-associated LFA-1, CD2 and LFA-3 molecules: cell adhesion of the immune system. Annu Rev Immunol 5: 223–242
Streuli M, Hall LR, Saga Y, Schlossman SF, Saito H (1987) Differential use of three exons generates at least five different mRNAs encoding human leucocyte common antigens. J Exp Med 166: 1548–1467
Tedder TF, Clement LT, Cooper MD (1985) Human lymphocyte differentiation antigens HB-10 and HB-11. II Differential production of B cell growth and differentiation factors by distinct helper T cell subpopulations. J Immunol 134: 2983–2988
Tighe H, Clark M, Waldmann H (1987) Blocking of cytotoxic T cell function by monoclonal antibodies against the CD45 antigen (T200/Leukocyte-common) antigen. Transplantation 44: 818–823
Yamada H, Martin PJ, Bean MA, Braun MP, Beatty PG, Sadamoto K, Hansen JA (1985) Monoclonal antibody 9.3 and anti-CD11 antibodies define reciprocal subsets of lymphocytes. Eur J Immunol 15: 1164–1168

# Suppressor T-Cell Memory

S. Adelstein, H. Pritchard-Briscoe, R. H. Loblay and A. Basten



## 1 Introduction

The immune response of the host to its environment necessitates a finely tuned network of feedback mechanisms designed to provide for an effective humoral and cellular response to potential pathogens without damage to self tissues. Therefore the maintenance of the immunological *milieu interieur* depends not only on counterbalances to regulate the extent of protective immune responses to foreign antigens but also on a series of controls to limit potential self-reactivity. Among the cybernetic mechanisms thought to be responsible for immuno regulation are antigen itself, antibody-mediated feedback, T-cell-dependent suppression and idiotypic networks (Basten et al. 1980; Nossal 1983).

The efficiency of the adaptive immune system depends on generation of memory as well as effector lymphocytes with specificity for foreign antigens. In collaborative antibody responses, the development of memory has been docu-

Clinical Immunology Research Centre, University of Sydney, Sydney, Australia

Current Topics in Microbiology and Immunology, Vol. 159

mented in both T-helper and B-cell lineages (Miller and Sprent 1971), while in cell-mediated reactions such as delayed hypersensitivity, allograft rejection and cytotoxicity, memory is a property of the T-cell subsets mediating each type of response (see other chapters in this volume). In this context memory can be defined as the capacity of the immune system, upon re-exposure to a previously encountered antigen, to mount an accelerated, augmented, and more prolonged response than after the primary stimulus. If such secondary responses are to be effectively controlled it would be expected, on a priori grounds, that regulatory mechanisms involving suppressor T cells would also exhibit anamnestic responses. Furthermore, if suppressor memory could be selectively induced early in ontogeny as a result of exposure to self-antigens, an important role could be envisaged for such cells in the maintenance of self-tolerance.

The aim of this review is to present evidence demonstrating the existence of suppressor T-cell memory and its importance in regulation and tolerance. The experiments described are consistent with the hypothesis that:

(a) exposure to antigen normally leads to concomitant activation of T cells with helper and suppressor function which can be distinguished by a number of criteria;
(b) cells mediating suppressor activity exist in two distinct physiological states, i.e., as short-lived effector cells and long-lived memory cells; and
(c) in contrast to memory helper cells, the cells responsible for memory (secondary) suppression exist in a functionally quiescent state until reactivated by exposure to antigen.

The potency of secondary suppression as observed in the experiments outlined below leaves little room for doubt about the existence of suppressor T cells as a distinct functional subset (Möller 1988), although much remains to be learned about their origins, their functional and phenotypic properties, and their relationships to and interactions with other T-cell subsets.

## 2 Demonstration of Suppressor Memory

Effector cells with suppressor activity have been demonstrated in many experimental models of immunoregulation and tolerance (Basten et al. 1980; Flood 1985). To test for the existence of suppressor memory, the antigen human gammaglobulin (HGG) was used since it can be presented to the immune system in either immunogenic (aggregated, aHGG) or tolerogenic (deaggregated, dHGG) form and has been shown to induce T cells with helper or suppressor function (Basten et al. 1975; Benjamin 1975; Doyle et al. 1976). CBA/Ca/T6 mice were immunised with aHGG and their spleen cells were transferred at day 10 into irradiated recipients together with hapten (dinitrophenyl; DNP)-primed and carrier (HGG)-primed cells. Controls received either no putative suppressor cells or a comparable number of spleen cells from unimmunised donors. On challenge with DNP-HGG, antigen-specific suppression of the collaborative antibody response was observed 7 days later and was shown to be mediated by a population of cells expressing Thy-1 (i.e., Thy-1$^+$ cells) which also express CD8 (Ly-2) and the serologically defined I-J determinant, but not CD4 (L3T4). The development of suppressor memory in mice given aHGG was examined by challenging them with HGG in tolerogenic form 4 or more weeks after primary immunisation. dHGG was used because of its known capacity to exert a preferential effect on T-cell-mediated suppression without activating T-helper cells (Basten et al. 1978). When the suppressor activity of spleen cells from these mice was compared with the 'primary' suppressive effects of cells obtained from mice given aHGG 10 days previously, significantly greater inhibition of the anti-hapten response was observed (Loblay et al. 1978). In additional experiments 'secondary' suppression was shown (a) to occur more rapidly, (b) to be induced by lower numbers of cells (Fig. 1) and (c) to be longer lasting than the primary suppressor response. In view of the presence of high levels of anti-HGG antibodies in the pre-immunised donors and the known importance of immune complexes in regulation of immune responses, it was necessary to exclude a role for them in the augmented secondary suppressor response. Normal mice were

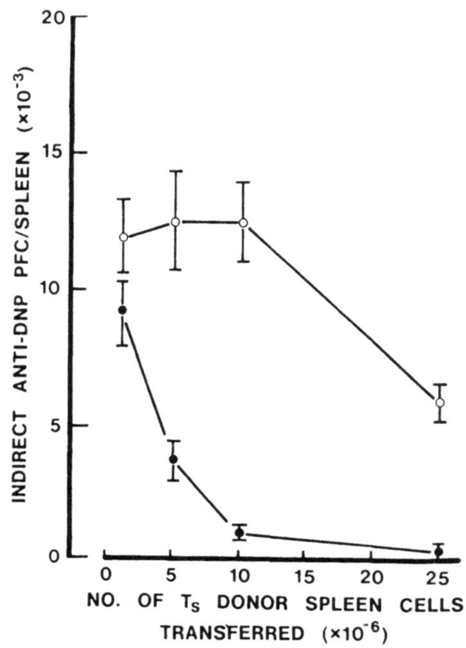


**Fig. 1** Comparison of potency of 'primary' and 'secondary' suppressor cells. Normal mice (○) or mice immunized with aHGG 8 weeks previously (●) were given 3 mg dHGG intraperitoneally. Then cells were collected on day 7 and varying numbers transferred into groups of six irradiated (750 R) recipients. Each recipient was then given $5 \times 10^6$ DNP-primed and $5 \times 10^6$ HGG-primed spleen cells together with 500 $\mu$g $DNP_{10}HGG$. Indirect splenic anti-DNP PFC responses were assayed 7 days later. PFC = plaque farming cells. [Reproduced with permission of the authors and publishers from Loblay et al. (1984), p. 17]

given large amounts of purified anti-HGG antibodies followed by a standard dose of dHGG 24 h later and their spleen cells assayed for suppression as described above. No augmentation of suppression occurred, thereby indicating that antibody-mediated feedback was not responsible for the secondary suppressor effect (LOBLAY et al. 1978). The results therefore provided convincing evidence for the existence of suppressor memory.

Reactivation of suppressor function has also been studied by EARDLEY and SERCARZ (1977), who showed recall of specific suppression in vitro; however, the response lacked the secondary augmentation characteristic of memory, presumably because the investigators boosted with antigen in immunogenic rather than tolerogenic form which would have led to simultaneous activation of memory T-helper cells.

## 3 Characteristics of Suppressor Memory

In contrast to helper T-cell memory, secondary suppression was only demonstrable after re-exposure of the animal to antigen, prior to adoptive transfer. This suggested that the memory-bearing cells exist in a functionally quiescent or 'silent' state until they experience a secondary antigenic stimulus which leads to the accelerated reappearance of effector cells. The distinction between memory and effector cell function was most clearly demonstrable after priming with low doses of dHGG. A single dose of 100 μg dHGG was insufficient to generate detectable primary suppression; however, an anamnestic secondary suppressor response could be elicited by aHGG challenge after a single injection of as little as 1–10 μg of deaggregated antigen, indicating that the latter had been effective in inducing suppressor T-cell ($T_s$) memory (LOBLAY et al. 1983). The requirement for restimulation with antigen before testing for secondary suppressor effector function may explain why the presence of suppressor memory has been overlooked in some experimental systems where assays for suppression were carried out without a prior antigen boost (PARKS et al. 1979).

Suppressor memory is extremely long-lived. According to experiments carried out in both immune and tolerant mice, the life-span of memory-bearing suppressor cells in the HGG system exceeds 150 days (LOBLAY et al. 1983, 1984). Keyhole limpet haemocyanin (KLH)-specific memory suppressor cells of comparable longevity have been reported by KANELLOPOULOS-LANGEVIN et al. (1984). By contrast, effectors of primary suppression have a lifespan of between 30 and 40 days (LOBLAY et al. 1984). In addition, it has been shown that suppressor memory can be induced by antenatal exposure to HGG via the placenta (FAZEKAS de St. GROTH et al. 1984) and is preserved in aging mice after memory in the helper cell and B-cell lineages has waned (CALLARD et al. 1980). These findings support a role for memory suppression in regulation of immune responses including those to self-antigens throughout life.

## 4 Induction of Suppressor Memory and Effector Cells

The cell interactions involved in memory and effector cell induction could not be studied in mixing experiments because of the presence of non-specific inhibition of responses in double adoptive transfer experiments (LOBLAY, unpublished observations). An alternative strategy was to deplete various cell populations in vivo by injection of anti-T-cell subset antibodies at various times in relation to challenge with antigen using the HGG system described above. Induction of secondary suppression was dependent on the interaction between two distinct Thy-1$^+$ T-cell populations, i.e., the Ly-1$^+$ (CD1), Ly-2$^-$ (CD8), L3T4$^-$ (CD4), IJ$^+$ population with suppressor inducer/amplifier function and the Ly-1$^-$ Ly-2$^+$ L3T4$^-$I-J$^+$ population[1] with suppressor effector function (PRITCHARD-BRISCOE, unpublished observations). The quiescent memory-bearing cells themselves displayed the same phenotype as these suppressor inducers, namely Ly-1$^+$ I-J$^+$ but Ly-2$^-$ L3T4$^-$. The lack of either of the cell interaction molecules normally required for optimal T-cell activation provides an attractive explanation for the quiescent nature of the memory suppressor cell, in contrast to the T-helper memory cell which expresses a high density of CD4. Further evidence in favour of the categorisation of memory suppressor cells within the double-negative T-cell subset in the periphery comes from experiments demonstrating that Ly-1$^+$ double-negative T-cell clones, irrespective of the I-J status, are potent inducers of suppression (HODES 1985). Alternatively, re-exposure of memory suppressor cells to antigen could lead to expression of Ly-2 and differentiation into Ly-2$^+$ effectors of suppression. Although theoretically feasible, there are no data to support an obligatory role for CD8 in the expression of suppressor responses; indeed, the lack of evidence of major histocompatibility complex (MHC) restriction of suppressor function would argue against such a possibility (H. PRITCHARD-BRISCOE, R. LOBLAY and A. BASTEN, unpublished observations).

The use of I-J as a cell marker for suppressor cells has been criticised on the grounds that no class II MHC locus can be assigned to I-J by serological analysis (STEINMETZ et al. 1982) and I-J$^+$ suppressor hybridomas lack any mRNA hybridising with class II DNA (KRONENBERG et al. 1983). Nevertheless, antibodies to I-J are highly effective in vivo and in vitro in abrogating suppressor function without influencing cytotoxic or helper activity (BASTEN et al. 1978) and are therefore a valuable tool for analysing the cell interactions involved in regulation of immune responses.

From the above experiments it is possible to formulate two alternative (though not mutually exclusive) models of the induction pathways for suppressor memory and effector cells (Fig. 2). One possibility is that the quiescent memory

---

[1] Ly-1$^-$ refers to phenotype as determined by in vivo and/or in vitro depletion experiments. T cells which are dull Ly-1 staining on fluorescence-activated cell sorter (FACS) analysis are not depleted by these procedures

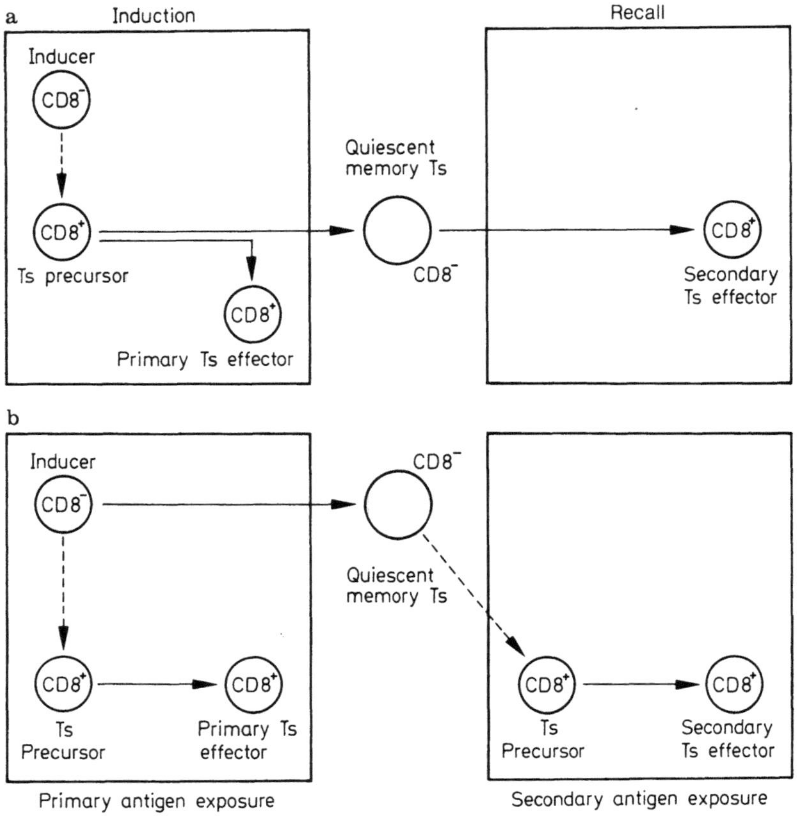


**Fig. 2 a, b.** Two alternative models of the induction pathways for memory suppressor cells (*Ts*). **a** The quiescent memory suppressor cell is derived from the same virgin precursor cell as the primary effector cell and may differentiate into secondary effector cells. **b** Memory is carried by the suppressor inducer cell distinct from the precursors of suppressor effector cell. *Solid lines* indicate a differentiation sequence; *broken lines* indicate an induction process.

cells are derived from the same precursors as those which give rise to primary suppressor effector cells (Fig. 2a). The memory cells would then differentiate into secondary suppressor effector cells in response to antigen re-exposure, possibly also forming new memory cells. As mentioned previously, the sequential functional changes from precursor to memory to effector cells would be accompanied by a loss and then reappearance, successively, of surface CD8 molecules. An alternative interpretation of the above findings is shown in Fig. 2b. Here it is envisaged that memory is carried by the inducer population, with primary and secondary suppressor effector cells arising from a common pool of suppressor precursor cells which have not previously encountered antigen. These virgin precursor cells would be capable of terminal differentiation into short-lived effector cells, but not into long-lived memory cells.

## 5 Role of Memory Suppression in Regulation of Immune Responses

Little is known of the precise mechanism(s) whereby suppressor effector cells exert their inhibitory actions, although it has been suggested that they may do so via release of 'suppressor factors' (GREEN et al. 1983). Our own data indicate that activated suppressor cells must be present during the first 24 h after antigenic stimulation in order to effectively inhibit an adoptive hapten-carrier response, and that under these circumstances suppression is dominant, i.e. suppressed target cells cannot be activated by exposure to a large excess of available helper cells (LOBLAY, unpublished observations). These observations, together with the rapid onset and potency of secondary suppression (Fig. 1), raise the interesting question of how the immune system manages to mount any secondary responses at all in the face of suppressor memory (LOBLAY and BASTEN 1986). The likely answer comes from studies of the kinetics of suppressor and helper activity in the primary and secondary responses to HGG (LOBLAY et al. 1984). Virgin and primed mice were immunised with HGG in aggregated or soluble form respectively, and at various intervals thereafter spleen cells were assayed for help and suppression in an adoptive anti-hapten response (Fig. 3). In the primary response (open circles) an early burst of helper activity occurred which reached a peak on day 3 after immunisation and was then followed by onset of suppression.

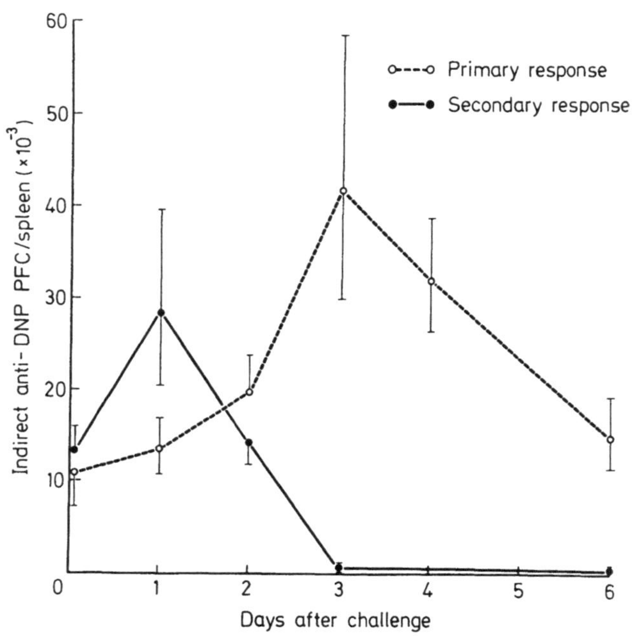


**Fig. 3.** Accelerated induction kinetics of help and suppression in the primary (*open circles*) versus secondary (*closed circles*) response to aHGG. Each point represents the geometric mean of anti-DNP PFC spleen ± SE from groups of six irradiated recipients

By contrast, in the secondary response (closed circles) the burst of help occurred earlier (i.e. on day 1) and by day 3 the anti-hapten response was completely suppressed. Thus, the existence of memory for suppression as well as help was confirmed in primed hosts. Furthermore, the results indicate that helper cells are activated more rapidly than suppressors, thereby allowing high-affinity B cells to escape and generate the secondary antibody response. On the other hand, these data do not tell us whether help and suppression is carried by the same or different T-cell populations. To study this, spleen cells from HGG-primed mice were treated with anti-Ia and complement 3 days after boosting with antigen (i.e. at the peak of suppression) and assayed for help and suppression in the usual way. Under these circumstances suppression was completely abrogated while hlep became readily demonstrable (LOBLAY et al. 1984). Spleen cells from primed mice therefore contain two distinct subsets of T-cells, one capable of mediating memory for help and the other memory for suppression, which reinforces the concept that suppressor cells exist as a distinct subset and that suppression is not due to anti-idiotypic T cells cytotoxic to T-helper cells (HEUER et al. 1982).

## 6 Role of Suppressor Memory in Tolerance to Foreign Antigens

It is now generally accepted that T-cell-dependent suppression is important in regulation of immune responses to exogenous antigens (BASTEN et al. 1980), but its role in tolerance has been more controversial. Indeed, several lines of evidence from the HGG system have pointed to a clear-cut dissociation between tolerance and suppression. For example, suppression is demonstrable in adoptive transfer for only 30 to 40 days after tolerance induction, whereas the duration of tolerance in the intact animal is of the order of 100 days or more after a single dose of HGG in deaggregated form (BENJAMIN 1975; DOYLE et al. 1976). Secondly, tolerance but not suppression can be induced in nude mice (ETLINGER and CHILLER 1977). Thirdly, pretreatment with colchicine results in selective abrogation of suppression but does not affect the tolerant state (PARKS et al. 1979). In each situation, however, only a primary suppressor response was studied and memory suppression was ignored. When the latter is taken into account a much closer association between tolerance and suppression becomes apparent (LOBLAY et al. 1983).

The role of memory suppression in HGG tolerance was examined in parallel with helper activity. Following tolerance induction, no helper cells could be demonstrated, as expected, while a wave of primary suppression occurred which lasted for 30 to 40 days and then subsided. On boosting with HGG in tolerogenic form between days 60 and 135 (i.e. after the primary wave of suppression had waned) tolerance was maintained and more profound suppression was apparent. These findings are consistent with the generation of long-lived memory

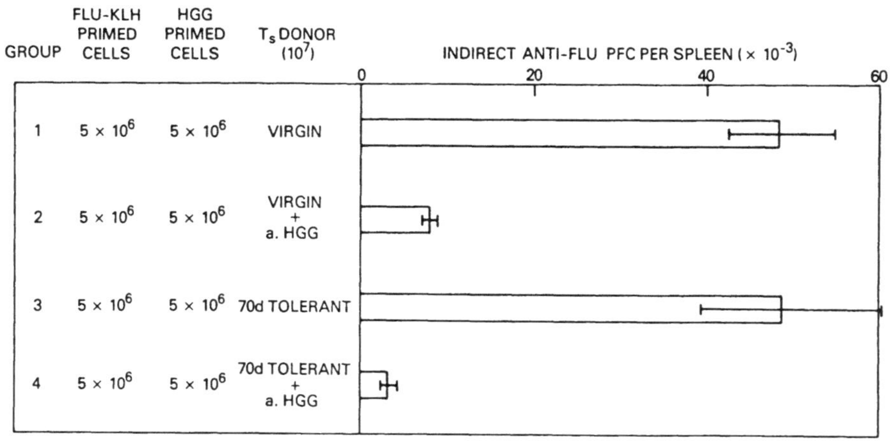


**Fig. 4.** Memory suppression in tolerant mice challenged with HGG in immunogenic form (aHGG). Note that no suppression occurred in tolerant mice not challenged with antigen (group 3). Each histogram represents the geometric mean PFC $\pm$ SE of 6 recipients per group. *FLU* = the hapten, fluorescein. [Reproduced from LOBLAY et al. (1983), p 901 by copyright permission of the Rockefeller University Press and with permission of the authors]

suppressor cells during initial tolerance induction, the lifespan of which parallels the duration of tolerance. Similar results were obtained when the tolerant mice were challenged with HGG in immunogenic form (Fig. 4). Since this is the usual way of testing for unresponsiveness in tolerance, the data strongly support a major role for memory cells, but not for the shorter-lived effector suppressor cells in maintenance of the tolerant state. Further confirmation for such a conclusion comes from (a) the demonstration of memory suppression in nude mice which are known to contain small numbers of T cells (BASTEN et al. 1985); (b) the fact that, in contrast to primary suppression, memory suppression like tolerance is resistant to colchicine treatment (CRESWICK and BASTEN, unpublished observations); and (c) the fact that low doses of HGG can induce memory suppression as well as tolerance in the absence of primary suppression (LOBLAY et al. 1983). Interestingly, the lifespan of suppressor effectors is the same as the duration of tolerance to HGG in the B-cell compartment, while memory suppression is of comparable longevity to tolerance in both the T-cell compartment and at the level of the whole animal (WEIGLE 1973). This finding is consistent with a direct effect of suppressor cells on the B cell.

# 7 Role of Memory Suppression in Tolerance to Self-Antigens

## 7.1 Model Involving Antigen Exposure In Utero

T-cell-dependent suppression specific for self-antigens has been documented in a number of models of autoimmunity (BASTEN et al. 1980; GIBSON et al. 1985) and

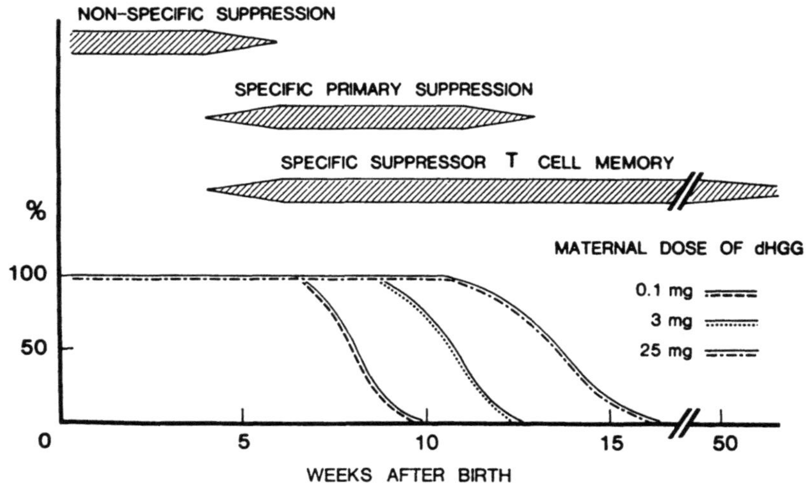


**Fig. 5.** Schematic diagram of tolerance and suppression after prenatal administration of dHGG. The duration of tolerance was dose-dependent whereas that of suppression was not. [Reproduced with permission of the authors and publishers from FAZEKAS DE ST. GROTH et al. (1984), p. 234]

has been taken as a priori evidence for involvement of suppressor cells at least as a fail-safe mechanism in maintenance of self-tolerance. The case in favour of a role for suppression in self-tolerance would be strengthened if exposure to antigen during ontogeny could be formally shown to lead to generation of long-lived memory-bearing suppressor cells.

To examine this proposition, use was made of the fact that HGG can be transferred across the placenta of mice from mother to offspring, so that it is handled by the developing immune system as if it were 'self' (FAZEKAS DE ST. GROTH et al. 1984). Following exposure to HGG in utero, tolerance was demonstrable in offspring for between 7 and 8 weeks postnatally depending on the dose of antigen used (Fig. 5). Primary suppression and suppressor memory were assayed in adoptive transfer as described previously. Up to 5 weeks of age, suppression proved to be non-specific, but thereafter specific inhibition of anti-hapten antibody production could be detected—for 3 months in the case of primary suppression and for over 6 months in the case of memory suppression. The lack of correlation between the kinetics of tolerance and those of suppression appears at first sight to argue against a role for memory-bearing suppressor cells in the maintenance of tolerance. However, it should be recalled that the levels of self-antigen (HGG) would have declined rapidly after birth at the same time as the number of immunocompetent B cells increased. Thus, to mimic natural self-tolerance more precisely, repeated injections of HGG should have been given. Indeed, when this procedure was adopted by WATERS et al. (1979), antenatal tolerance to HGG was prolonged for up to 50 weeks. Taken together, these data are consistent with the hypothesis that the maintenance of self-tolerance involves memory suppression provided antigen is continuously present.

## 7.2 Red Cell Model

The disadvantage of using exogenous antigens to mimic self is that they may not be presented to the immune system in association with class I MHC antigens (TOWNSEND et al. 1986). Evidence was therefore sought for the existence of memory suppression in a model of natural self-tolerance. The model chosen was one involving self-tolerance to autologous mouse red cells (MRBC). In this system it is possible to demonstrate selective suppression of the auto-antibody response to mouse red cells following challenge with cross-reactive rat erythrocytes (PLAYFAIR and MARSHALL-CLARKE 1973; COX and HOWLES 1981). The cells responsible carry I-J as they do in the HGG system (GIBSON et al. 1985). It was postulated that, if suppressor memory is intimately involved in self-tolerance to red blood cells, depletion of suppressor precursors during ontogeny should result in an increased susceptibility to autoimmune haemolysis. This hypothesis was tested by repeatedly immunising B10.A(3R) female mice with B10.A(5R) cells to produce circulating anti-I-J antibodies of $H\text{-}2^k$ specificity. The B10.A(3R) females were then mated with CBA ($H\text{-}2^k$) males so that the resulting F1 progeny were exposed to maternal anti-$I\text{-}J^k$ antibodies throughout gestation. On challenging the anti-I-J antibody-treated offspring with rat red blood cells (RRBC) in adult life, a higher auto-antibody response was observed than in age-matched controls (Fig. 6). By contrast, there was no difference in antibody production to foreign determinants on RRBC (GIBSON et al. 1985). Furthermore, if the same F1 mice were repeatedly injected with anti-I-J sera postnatally and thymectomised at 4 weeks of age to prevent replenishment of the suppressor cell pool, more than half of them spontaneously developed auto-antibodies not only to red cells but to other auto-antigens (e.g. nuclear antigens) as well. In other words, depletion of $I\text{-}J^+$ suppressor cells, including those with memory-bearing potential, early in development resulted in a loss of self-tolerance, as indicated by the enhanced auto-antibody response (KATEKAR and BASTEN, unpublished observations).

Two groups of experiments pointed to the self-reactive B cell as the target of memory suppression. In the first, the specificity profiles of B-cell hybridomas obtained by fusion of spleen cells from anti-I-J-exposed and control mice with the NS-1 cell line were compared. The specificity of hybridomas derived from the controls was restricted to foreign (anti-RRBC) and cross-reactive epitopes only, whereas in the case of hybridomas from the depleted mice the relative proportion of cross-reactive clones increased and a number of self-reactive clones appeared (WALKER et al. 1987). In the second experiment, the proliferative response of RRBC-primed lymph node cells from anti-I-J-exposed and control mice was measured in the presence of MRBC or RRBC. Although there was some increase in proliferation of T cells to RRBC from the suppressor cell-depleted mice, the

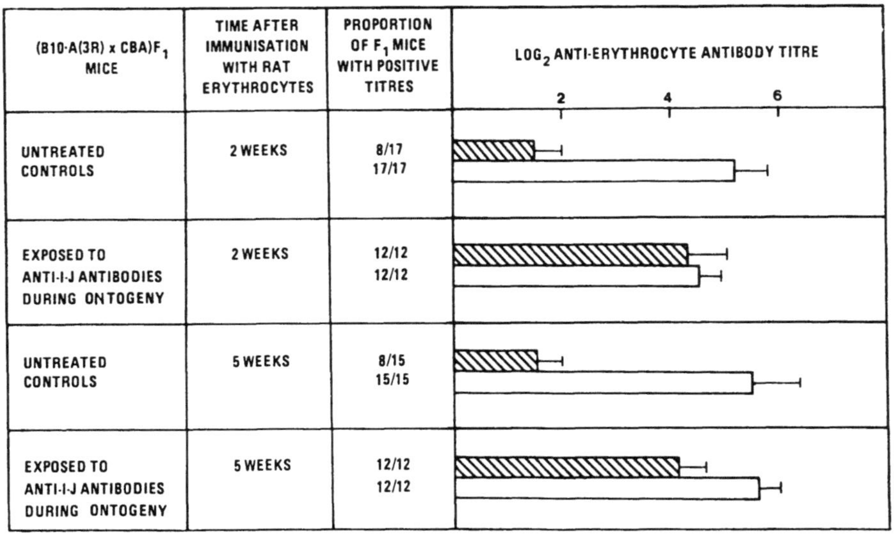


**Fig. 6.** Comparison of anti-MRBC (*hatched bars*) and anti-RRBC (*open bars*) antibody responses in [B10.A(3R) × CBA] F1 mice exposed to maternal anti-I-J antibodies during ontogeny and normal F1 controls. The anti-MRBC response was measured by the direct anti-globulin test and the anti-RRBC response by indirect haemagglutination. The difference in anti-MRBC titres was significant at both time points whereas the anti-RRBC titres were similar. [Reproduced with permission of the authors and publisher from Gibson et al. (1985), p 5150]

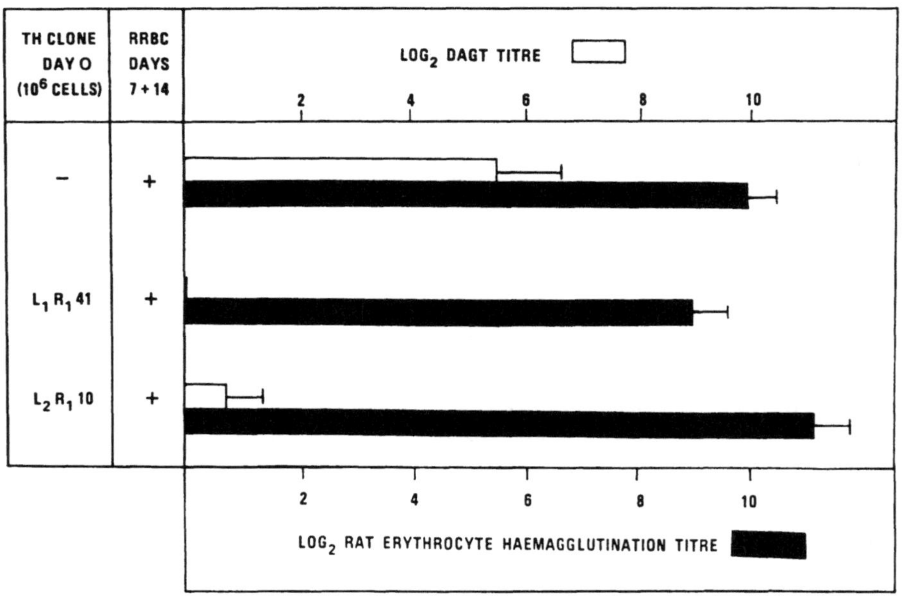


**Fig. 7.** Selective suppression of the anti-MRBC antibody response in normal mice given $10^6$ cells from two long-term cross-reactive T-cell lines. At the time of transfer the T cells did not express Ly-2 or L3T4 and were not actively proliferating. [Reproduced from Gibson (1986)]

minimal anti-self response observed in the control lymph node cells was not affected by prior exposure to anti-I-J antibodies in utero (GIBSON et al. 1985).

The overall conclusion from these experiments is that exposure to self-antigens such as MRBC leads to deletion of self-specific T-helper cells and to generation of a long-lived pool of memory suppressor cells which on reactivation by exposure to cross-reactive antigens maintain the tolerant state through down regulation of self-specific B cells. Confirmation of this conclusion was obtained by injecting normal mice with either of two interleukin-2 (IL-2)-dependent T-cell clones ($10^6$ cells per recipient) cross-reactive to MRBC and RRBC (GIBSON and BASTEN 1988). As shown in Fig. 7, profound inhibition of auto-antibody production occurred whereas the response to foreign epitopes on RRBC was unaffected. When spleen cells were transferred from these mice into a second set of recipients, selective suppression of the anti-self response was again observed, indicating that the effect was mediated by activation of pre-existing self-specific memory suppressor cells (GIBSON and BASTEN, unpublished observations). Interestingly, the T-cell clones lacked both Ly-2 and L3T4 at the time when the transfer experiments were carried out.

## 7.3 Transplacental Traffic

Evidence has also been obtained which suggests that memory suppressor cells, but not memory T-helper cells, can be transferred from mother to offspring via the placenta. For this purpose female CBA mice were immunised with HGG in immunogenic form at 6 weeks of age to generate memory for both help and suppression. After a further 12 weeks they were bred with BALB/c males which differ at the Ly-2(CD8) locus. When the F1 offspring were 8 weeks old, their spleen cells were assayed for help and suppression in an adoptive anti-hapten antibody response. No help was demonstrable, whereas clear evidence for memory suppression was obtained after a boost with soluble antigen (Fig. 8; group 5 versus group 2). Furthermore, suppression was reversed by pretreatment of the spleen cells with complement plus anti-Ly-2 antibodies directed to the maternal (Ly-2.1) but not the paternal (Ly-2.2) haplotype (group 6 versus group 7). No evidence for transfer of antigen across the placenta was obtained; in other words secondary suppression in the F1 offspring was mediated by long-lived Ly-$2^+$ T cells from the mother (K.L. WONG, R. LOBLAY and A. BASTEN, unpublished observations). The susceptibility of the suppressor cells of maternal origin to anti-Ly-2 antibody could have resulted from the acquisition of CD8 after restimulation with antigen and is consistent with the suggestion mentioned previously that the double-negative memory-bearing suppressors may be the precursors of $CD8^+$ effector cells.

A similar conclusion was reached in the red cell model described above. RRBC-immunised CBA females (I-$J^k$) were mated with normal C57BL6 males (I-$J^b$) and the spleen cells from the F1 offspring assayed for suppression in adult life. Potent secondary suppression was again demonstrable, which was completely

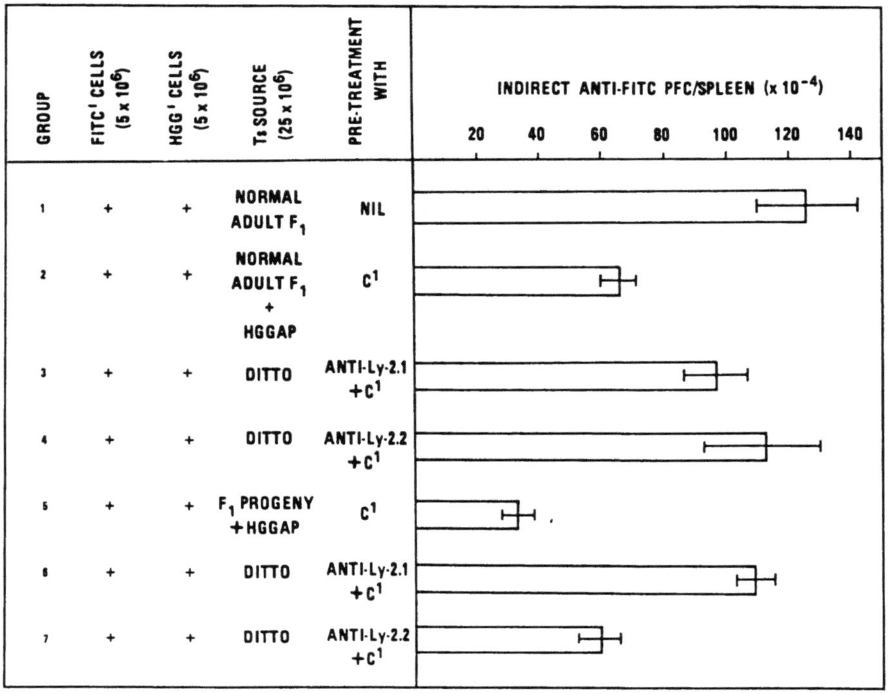


**Fig. 8.** Maternal origin of memory suppressor cells in the [BALB/c × CBA]F1 offspring of long-term HGG-primed CBA females. Antibodies to CD8 (alleles Ly-2.1 and Ly-2.2) reversed suppression to F1 spleen cells (groups 3 and 4), whereas only anti-Ly-2.1 directed to the maternal haplotype did so in the case of F1 progeny of HGG-primed mothers (groups 6 versus 7) FITC = Fluorescein; C′ = Guinea pig complement; HGGAP = primed and boosted with HGG

reversed by pretreatment with complement and anti-I-J$^k$ but not anti-I-J$^b$ antibodies (GIBSON and BASTEN 1988), once again pointing to transplacental passage of memory-bearing suppressor cells. The phenotype of the cells passing from mother to offspring could not be studied directly by FACS analysis due to the low numbers involved.

The significance of the apparently preferential traffic of suppressor memory across the placenta is not clear. However, one attractive hypothesis is that such cells may play a part in the induction of self-tolerance, and possibly in selective processes involved in shaping the T-cell repertoire.

# 8 Conclusions

It is clear that the phenomenon of memory suppression exists and that it is important in regulation of immune responses to foreign antigens. Memory suppression also appears to be involved in tolerance, although its precise role during induction versus maintenance requires further definition. In particular, it will be necessary to determine whether suppressor signals can be stored by target cells for significant periods of time, to elucidate the nature of the serologically defined I-J determinant and to define the functional significance of double-negative and $\gamma\delta$-bearing T cells, both of which could in theory be responsible for the carriage of memory suppression. Indeed, this possibility is worth investigating for several reasons. First, the frequency of both double-negative and $\gamma\delta$-cells is sufficiently low to make them plausible candidates for mediating suppression. Secondly, $\gamma\delta$-cells are cells without an obvious function (reviewed by JANEWAY 1988), but their suppressor activity has yet to be examined. Thirdly, $\gamma\delta$-cells do not appear to recognise class I or II MHC gene products even though some of them express CD8; on the other hand they may interact with class IB MHC-like molecules (KLEIN 1986; MATIS 1987) which could explain why suppression does not appear to be MHC restricted in the classical sense. Finally, the surveillance function postulated for $\gamma\delta$-cells (JANEWAY et al. 1988) could be one of suppression (rather than cytotoxicity) designed to minimise tissue damage on exposure to extrinsic antigens. This alternative is consistent with the recent suggestion by PEREIRA et al. (1988) that normal hosts contain functional suppressor but no cytolytic effector cells.

## References


Basten A, Miller JFAP, Johnson P (1975) T cell-dependent suppression of an anti-hapten antibody response. Transplant Rev 26: 130–169

Basten A, Miller JFAP, Loblay R, Johnson P, Gamble J, Chia E, Pritchard-Briscoe H, Callard R, McKenzie IFC (1978) T cell-dependent suppression of antibody production I. Characteristics of suppressor T cells following tolerance induction. Eur J Immunol 8: 360–370

Basten A, Loblay RH, Trent RJ, Gatenby PA (1980) Suppressor T cells in immune homeostasis. In: Thompson RA (ed) Recent advances in clinical immunology, vol 2. Churchill Livingstone Edinburgh, pp 33–63

Basten A, Gibson J, Loblay RH, Wong KL, Fazekas De St. Groth B (1985) The role of memory suppressor T cells in self tolerance: induction in utero and in athymic mice. Adv Exp Med Biol 186: 511–520

Benjamin DC (1975) Evidence for specific suppression in the maintenance of immunologic tolerance. J Exp Med 141: 635–646

Callard RE, Fazekas de St. Groth B, Basten A, McKenzie IFC (1980) Immune function in aged mice V. Role of suppressor cells. J Immunol 124: 52–58

Cox KO, Howles A (1981) Induction and regulation of autoimmune haemolytic anaemia in a mouse model. Immunol Rev 55: 394–401

Doyle MV, Parks DE, Weigle WO (1976) Specific transient suppression of the immune response by HGG tolerant spleen cells II. Effector cells and target cells. J Immunol 117: 1152–1158

Eardley DD, Sercarz EE (1977) Recall of specific suppression: co-dominance of suppression after primary or secondary antigen stimulation. J Immunol 118: 1306–1310

Etlinger HM, Chiller JM (1977) Induction of tolerance in athymic mice with an antigen which is highly immunogenic in euthymic mice. Cell Immunol 33: 297–308

Fazekas de St. Groth B, Basten A, Loblay RH (1984) Induction of memory and effector suppressor T cells by perinatal exposure to antigen. Eur J Immunol 14: 228–235

Flood PM (1985) The role of suppressor cells in maintaining tolerance to self molecules—a commentary. J Mol Cell Immunol 2: 140–142

Gibson J, Basten A, Walker KZ, Loblay RH (1985) A role for suppressor T cells in induction of self-tolerance. Proc Natl Acad Sci USA 82: 5150–5154
Gibson J (1986) Mechanisms of self tolerance. PhD thesis, University of Sydney
Gibson J, Basten A (1988) In vivo properties of murine autoreactive T cell clones with specificity for erythrocytes. Autoimmunity 2, 21–29
Green DR, Flood PM and Gershon RK (1983) Immunoregulatory T-cell pathways. Annu Rev Immunol 1: 439–463
Heuer J, Bruner K, Opalka B, Kölsch E (1982) A cloned T-cell line from a tolerant mouse represents a novel antigen-specific suppressor cell type. Nature 296: 456–459
Hodes RJ (1985) Cloned Lyt-$1^+$, $2^-$ T suppressor cells—a commentary. J Mol Cell Immunol 2: 14–16
Janeway CA (1988) Frontiers of the immune system. Nature 333: 804–806
Janeway CA, Jones B, Hayday A (1988) Specificity and function of T cells bearing $\gamma\delta$ receptors. Immunol Today 9:3: 73–76
Kanellopoulos-Langevin C, Mathieson BJ, Perkins A, Maynard A, Asofsky R (1984) Regulation of anti-hapten responses *in vivo*: memory, carrier-specific Lyt-$2^+$ T cells can terminate antibody production without altering the peak of response. J Immunol 132:4: 1639–1646
Klein J (1986) Natural History of the Major Histocompatibility Complex. Wiley, New York
Kronenberg M, Steinmetz M, Kobon J, Kraig E, Kapp JA, Pierce CW, Sorensen CM, Suzuki G, Tada T, Hood L (1983) RNA transcript for I-J polypeptides are apparently not encoded between I-A and I-E subregions of the murine major histocompatibility complex. Proc Natl Acad Sci USA 80: 5704–5708
Loblay RH, Basten A (1986) Why is the immune system not overwhelmed by suppression? A reductionist paradox. In: Hoffman GW, Levy JG, Nepom GT (eds) Paradoxes in immunology. CRC Press, Boca Raton, FL, pp 115–120
Loblay RH, Pritchard-Briscoe H, Basten A (1978) Suppressor T cell memory. Nature 272: 620–622
Loblay RH, Fazekas de St. Groth B, Pritchard-Briscoe H, Basten A (1983) Suppressor T cell memory II: the role of memory suppressor T cells in tolerance to human gammaglobulin. J Exp Med 157: 957–973
Loblay RH, Pritchard-Briscoe H, Basten A (1984) Suppressor T cell memory: induction and recall of HGG-specific memory suppressor T cells and their role in regulation of antibody production. Aust J Exp Biol Med Sci 62: 11–25
Matis LA, Cron R, Bluestone JA (1987) Major histocompatibility complex-linked specificity of $\gamma\delta$ receptor bearing T lymphocytes. Nature 330: 262–64
Miller JFAP, Sprent J (1971) Cell-to-cell interaction in the immune response VI. Contribution of thymus-derived cells and antibody-forming cell precursors to immunological memory. J Exp Med 134: 66–82
Möller G (1988) Do suppressor T cells exist? Scand J Immunol 27: 247–250 (editorial)
Nossal GJV (1983) Cellular mechanisms of immunologic tolerance. Annu Rev Immunol 1: 33–62
Parks DE, Shaller DA, Weigle WO (1979) Induction and mode of action of suppressor cells generated against human gammaglobulin II. Effects of colchicine. J Exp Med 149: 1168–1182
Pereira P, Larsson-Sciard EL, Coutinho A, Bandeira A (1988) Suppressor versus cytotoxic CD$8^+$ T lymphocytes. Where are the artefacts? Scand J Immunol 27: 625–628
Playfair JHL, Marshall-Clarke S (1973) Induction of red cell auto-antibodies in normal mice. Nature (New Biology) 243: 213–214
Steinmetz M, Minard K, Horvath S, McNicholas J, Srelinger J, Wake C, Long E, Mach V, Hood L (1982) A molecular map of the immune response region from the major histocompatibility complex of the mouse. Nature 300: 35–42
Townsend ARM, Bastin J, Gould K, Brownlee GG (1986) Cytotoxic T lymphocytes recognize influenza haemagglutinin that lacks a signal sequence. Nature 324: 575–577
Walker KZ, Gibson J, Basten A (1987) Clonal analysis of autoreactive B cells in a murine model of autoimmune haemolytic anaemia. Cell Immunol 107: 227–237
Waters CA, Pilarski M, Wegman TG, Deiner E (1979) Tolerance induction during ontogeny I: presence of active suppression in mice rendered tolerant to human $\gamma$-globulin in utero correlated with the breakdown of the tolerant state. J Exp Med 149: 1134–1151
Weigle WO (1973) Immunological unresponsiveness. Adv Immunol 16: 61–122

# Subject Index

# Current Topics in Microbiology and Immunology

Volumes published since 1982 (and still available)

Vol. 100: **Boehmer, H. V.; Haas, W.; Köhler, G.; Melchers, F.; Zeuthen, J. (Ed.):** T Cell Hybridomas. A Workshop at the Basel Institute for Immunology. With the collaboration Buser-Boyd, S. 1982. 52 figs. XI, 262 pp. ISBN 3-540-11535-8

Vol. 101: **Graf, Thomas; Jaenisch, Rudolf (Ed.):** Tumorviruses, Neoplastic Transformation, and Differentiation. 1982. 27 figs. VIII, 198 pp. ISBN 3-540-11665-6

Vol. 106: **Vogt, Peter K.; Koprowski, Hilary (Ed.):** Mouse Mammary Tumor Virus. 1983. 12 figs. VII, 103 pp. ISBN 3-540-12828-X

Vol. 107: **Vogt, Peter K.; Koprowski; Hilary (Ed.):** Retroviruses 2. 1983. 26 figs. VII, 180 pp. ISBN 3-540-12384-9

Vol. 109: **Doerfler, Walter (Ed.):** The Molecular Biology of Adenoviruses 1. 30 Years of Adenovirus Research 1953–1983. 1983. 69 figs. XII, 232 pp. ISBN 3-540-13034-9

Vol. 110: **Doerfler, Walter (Ed.):** The Molecular Biology of Adenoviruses 2. 30 Years of Adenovirus Research 1953–1983. 1984. 49 figs. VIII, 265 pp. ISBN 3-540-13127-2

Vol. 112: **Vogt, Peter K.; Koprowski, Hilary (Ed.):** Retroviruses 3. 1984. 19 figs. VII, 115 pp. ISBN 3-540-13307-0

Vol. 113: **Potter, Michael; Melchers, Fritz; Weigert, Martin (Ed.):** Oncogenes in B-Cell Neoplasia. Workshop at the National Cancer Institute, National Institutes of Health, Bethesda, MD March 5–7, 1984. 1984. 65 figs. XIII, 268 pp. ISBN 3-540-13597-9

Vol. 115: **Vogt, Peter K. (Ed.):** Human T-Cell Leukemia Virus. 1985. 74 figs. IX, 266 pp. ISBN 3-540-13963-X

Vol. 116: **Willis, Dawn B. (Ed.):** Iridoviridae. 1985. 65 figs. X, 173 pp. ISBN 3-540-15172-9

Vol. 122: **Potter, Michael (Ed.):** The BALB/c Mouse. Genetics and Immunology. 1985. 85 figs. XVI, 254 pp. ISBN 3-540-15834-0

Vol. 124: **Briles, David E. (Ed.):** Genetic Control of the Susceptibility to Bacterial Infection. 1986. 19 figs. XII, 175 pp. ISBN 3-540-16238-0

Vol. 125: **Wu, Henry C.; Tai, Phang C. (Ed.):** Protein Secretion and Export in Bacteria. 1986. 34 figs. X, 211 pp. ISBN 3-540-16593-2

Vol. 126: **Fleischer, Bernhard; Reimann, Jörg; Wagner, Hermann (Ed.):** Specificity and Function of Clonally Developing T-Cells. 1986. 60 figs. XV, 316 pp. ISBN 3-540-16501-0

Vol. 127: **Potter, Michael; Nadeau, Joseph H.; Cancro, Michael P. (Ed.):** The Wild Mouse in Immunology. 1986. 119 figs. XVI, 395 pp. ISBN 3-540-16657-2

Vol. 128: 1986. 12 figs. VII, 122 pp. ISBN 3-540-16621-1

Vol. 129: 1986. 43 figs., VII, 215 pp. ISBN 3-540-16834-6

Vol. 130: **Koprowski, Hilary; Melchers, Fritz (Ed.):** Peptides as Immunogens. 1986. 21 figs. X, 86 pp. ISBN 3-540-16892-3

Vol. 131: **Doerfler, Walter; Böhm, Petra (Ed.):** The Molecular Biology of Baculoviruses. 1986. 44 figs. VIII, 169 pp. ISBN 3-540-17073-1

Vol. 132: **Melchers, Fritz; Potter, Michael (Ed.):** Mechanisms in B-Cell Neoplasia. Workshop at the National Cancer Institute, National Institutes of Health, Bethesda, MD, USA, March 24–26, 1986. 1986. 156 figs. XII, 374 pp. ISBN 3-540-17048-0

Vol. 133: **Oldstone, Michael B. (Ed.):** Arenaviruses. Genes, Proteins, and Expression. 1987. 39 figs. VII, 116 pp. ISBN 3-540-17246-7

Vol. 134: **Oldstone, Michael B. (Ed.):** Arenaviruses. Biology and Immunotherapy. 1987. 33 figs. VII, 242 pp. ISBN 3-540-17322-6

Vol. 135: **Paige, Christopher J.; Gisler, Roland H. (Ed.):** Differentiation of B Lymphocytes. 1987. 25 figs. IX, 150 pp. ISBN 3-540-17470-2

Vol. 136: **Hobom, Gerd; Rott, Rudolf (Ed.):** The Molecular Biology of Bacterial Virus Systems. 1988. 20 figs. VII, 90 pp. ISBN 3-540-18513-5

Vol. 137: **Mock, Beverly; Potter, Michael (Ed.):** Genetics of Immunological Diseases. 1988. 88 figs. XI, 335 pp. ISBN 3-540-19253-0

Vol. 138: **Goebel, Werner (Ed.):** Intracellular Bacteria. 1988. 18 figs. IX, 179 pp. ISBN 3-540-50001-4

Vol. 139: **Clarke, Adrienne E.; Wilson, Ian A. (Ed.):** Carbohydrate-Protein Interaction. 1988. 35 figs. IX, 152 pp. ISBN 3-540-19378-2

Vol. 140: **Podack, Eckhard R. (Ed.):** Cytotoxic Effector Mechanisms. 1989. 24 figs. VIII, 126 pp. ISBN 3-540-50057-X

Vol. 141: **Potter, Michael; Melchers, Fritz (Ed.):** Mechanisms in B-Cell Neoplasia 1988. Workshop at the National Cancer Institute, National Institutes of Health, Bethesda, MD, USA, March 23–25, 1988. 1988. 122 figs. XIV, 340 pp. ISBN 3-540-50212-2

Vol. 142: **Schüpbach, Jörg:** Human Retrovirology. Facts and Concepts. 1989. 24 figs. 115 pp. ISBN 3-540-50455-9

Vol. 143: **Haase, Ashley T.; Oldstone, Michael B. A. (Ed.):** In Situ Hybridization. 1989. 33 figs. XII, 90 pp. ISBN 3-540-50761-2

Vol. 144: **Knippers, Rolf; Levine, A. J. (Ed.):** Transforming Proteins of DNA Tumor Viruses. 1989. 85 figs. XIV, 300 pp. ISBN 3-540-50909-7

Vol. 145: **Oldstone, Michael B. A. (Ed.):** Molecular Mimicry. Cross-Reactivity between Microbes and Host Proteins as a Cause of Autoimmunity. 1989. 28 figs. VII, 141 pp. ISBN 3-540-50929-1

Vol. 146: **Mestecky, Jiri; McGhee, Jerry (Ed.):** New Strategies for Oral Immunization. International Symposium at the University of Alabama at Birmingham and Molecular Engineering Associates, Inc. Birmingham, AL, USA, March 21–22, 1988. 1989. 22 figs. IX, 237 pp. ISBN 3-540-50841-4

Vol. 147: **Vogt, Peter K. (Ed.):** Oncogenes. Selected Reviews. 1989. 8 figs. VII, 172 pp. ISBN 3-540-51050-8

Vol. 148: **Vogt, Peter K. (Ed.):** Oncogenes and Retroviruses. Selected Reviews. 1989. XII, 134 pp. ISBN 3-540-51051-6

Vol. 149: **Shen-Ong, Grace L. C.; Potter, Michael; Copeland, Neal G. (Ed.):** Mechanisms in Myeloid Tumorigenesis. Workshop at the National Cancer Institute, National Institutes of Health, Bethesda, MD, USA, March 22, 1988. 1989. 42 figs. X, 172 pp. ISBN 3-540-50968-2

Vol. 150: **Jann, Klaus; Jann, Barbara (Ed.):** Bacterial Capsules. 1989. 33 figs. XII, 176 pp. ISBN 3-540-51049-4

Vol. 151: **Jann, Klaus; Jann, Barbara (Ed.):** Bacterial Adhesins. 1990. 23 figs. XII, 192 pp. ISBN 3-540-51052-4

Vol. 152: **Bosma, Melvin J.; Phillips, Robert A.; Schuler, Walter (Ed.):** The Scid Mouse. Characterization and Potential Uses. EMBO Workshop held at the Basel Institute for Immunology, Basel, Switzerland, February 20–22, 1989. 1989. 72 figs. XII, 263 pp. ISBN 3-540-51512-7

Vol. 153: **Lambris, John D. (Ed.):** The Third Component of Complement. Chemistry and Biology. 1989. 38 figs. X, 251 pp. ISBN 3-540-51513-5

Vol. 154: **McDougall, James K. (Ed.):** Cytomegaloviruses. 1990. 58 figs. IX, 286 pp. ISBN 3-540-51514-3

Vol. 155: **Kaufmann, Stefan H. E. (Ed.):** T-Cell Paradigms in Parasitic and Bacterial Infections. 1990. 24 figs. IX, 162 pp. ISBN 3-540-51515-1

Vol. 156: **Dyrberg, Thomas (Ed.):** The Role of Viruses and the Immune System in Diabetes Mellitus. 1990. 15 figs. XI, 142 pp. ISBN 3-540-51918-1

Vol 157: **Swanstrom, Ronald; Vogt, Peter K. (Ed.):** Retroviruses. Strategies of Replication. 1990. 40 figs. XII, 260 pp. ISBN 3-540-51895-9

Vol 158: **Muzyczka, Nicholas (Ed.):** Viral Expression Vectors. 1990. approx. 20 figs. approx. XII, 190 pp. ISBN 3-540-52431-2

MIX
Papier aus verantwortungsvollen Quellen
Paper from responsible sources
FSC® C105338

If you have any concerns about our products,
you can contact us on
**ProductSafety@springernature.com**

In case Publisher is established outside the EU,
the EU authorized representative is:
**Springer Nature Customer Service Center GmbH**
**Europaplatz 3, 69115 Heidelberg, Germany**

Printed by Libri Plureos GmbH
in Hamburg, Germany